ACCLAIM FOR
Michael Reed Gach's
ARTHRITIS RELIEF PROGRAM

"What is so exciting to me about *Arthritis Relief at Your Fingertips* is that Michael Gach describes methods that provide distressed patients with a powerful yet safe tool to help them move toward a healthier and more pain-free existence. The author's techniques may give those who suffer from a chronic arthritic condition some control over their own destiny while complementing more traditional forms of therapy. This is no small achievement. . . .

"*Arthritis Relief at Your Fingertips* gives the reader hands-on, practical suggestions for many types and stages of arthritic and rheumatic conditions. Acupressure offers relief with no risk and at the same time is inexpensive and easily integrated into one's life. Michael Gach's arthritis exercises are easy to learn and easy to do. I strongly recommend this book to sufferers of arthritis or related soft tissue rheumatic disorders who are not satisfied living with chronic pain."

—Murray C. Sokoloff, M.D.,
Rheumatologist
Assistant Clinical Professor of Medicine,
Stanford University Medical Center

"Offers new insight. . . . What is different about this book is the emphasis on acupressure, a natural therapy used by the Chinese for thousands of years."

—*New York Daily News*

"Gach provides the reader with several positive approaches to dealing with arthritis."

—*Publishers Weekly*

ARTHRITIS RELIEF AT YOUR FINGERTIPS

Your Guide to Easing Aches and Pains Without Drugs

MICHAEL REED GACH

WARNER BOOKS

A Time Warner Company

This book is not intended as a substitute for medical advice. The reader should regularly consult a physician or health care professional in matters relating to health and particularly in respect to any symptoms which may require diagnosis or medical attention.

Warner Books, Inc., 1271 Avenue of the Americas, New York, NY 10020

Ⓦ A Time Warner Company

Printed in the United States of America
First trade printing: July 1990
10 9 8 7

Library of Congress Cataloging-in-Publication Data

Gach, Michael Reed.
  Arthritis Relief at Your Fingertips
  Bibliography: p.
  Includes index.
  1. Arthritis — Physical therapy.   2. Arthritis — Exercise therapy.   3. Acupressure.
  4. Self-care.
  Health. I. Title.
  RC933.G32   1989   616.7'22
  ISBN 0-446-39156-5

Cover design by Jackie Seow

TABLE OF CONTENTS

FOREWORD I

What is so exciting to me about *Arthritis Relief at Your Fingertips* is that Michael Gach describes methods that provide distressed patients with a powerful yet safe tool to help them move toward a healthier and more pain free existence. The author's techniques may give those who suffer from a chronic arthritic condition some control over their own destiny while complementing more traditional forms of therapy. This is no small achievement.

People with illness who try to help themselves usually heal faster and more completely. That this occurs is well-known and acknowledged by the healing professions. Michael Gach's book offers patients with arthritis and related conditions a tool to do just that. Acupressure is not meant to replace traditional methods of medical treatment and in many cases may be used as a very beneficial supplement to these methods. Furthermore, in the treatment of the minor aches and pains we all experience, acupressure alone may be the method of therapy that is needed. Scientifically, it is difficult to know exactly how these acupressure techniques produce their benefit. After thousands of years of empirical application, the methods have survived because they work. Acupressure like acupuncture appears to relieve pain directly

through the release of natural painkilling chemicals (called endorphins) in the body and indirectly through the relaxation response.

I have personally experienced the tremendous power of acupressure and have used it in my practice. I believe many patients with arthritis or soft tissue rheumatism who regularly practice the self-help techniques outlined by Michael Gach can greatly benefit from the depth of relaxation that naturally results in decreased aches and pains. Many patients may also experience a deepening awareness that not only better enables them to attend to basic body signals, but helps them recognize and possibly change detrimental life patterns, coping mechanisms, and habits.

Deep relaxation naturally benefits many arthritic and related rheumatic conditions, including inflammatory, degenerative, and muscular types. Being calm promotes a feeling of well-being, just as being stressed makes everything seem worse.

Arthritis, like any serious illness, may often be a sign that one's life is out of balance and that changes need to be made. Arthritis and the related soft tissue rheumatic disorders could be nature's way of telling us to slow down a little and take care of ourselves. Instead of paying attention to this important natural signal, what most of us do is reach into the medicine cabinet for a quick fix. When that doesn't work we make an appointment with our physician or chiropractor.

After an appropriate evaluation, the physician or chiropractor will usually label the condition, based on the practitioner's training, experience, and the particular signs and symptoms presented by the patient. Treatment is often prescribed or administered by the practitioner. This usually includes prescription drugs when a physician is consulted, and manipulation in the case of the chiropractor. Often, little or no attempt is made to look for the underlying factors such as the ones alluded to above. While the drugs or manipulative techniques might relieve the condition, unless the underlying factors are recognized and addressed, the condition will in many cases not be cured, only palliated, and may recur.

What is the price one must pay for this quick fix? Drug side effects of varying severity are not only common, they may be serious in rare cases. In an age where natural is "in," it is amazing what many of us put into our bodies. Is it any wonder that the anti-arthritic, analgesic drug market is several billion dollars a year in the USA alone?

Although I often recommend aspirin or aspirin-like drugs to relieve arthritic pain, I am aware of the potential side effects of these drugs and take precautions to minimize them. I am well aware of the limitations of this form of therapy and in selected cases may add acupressure or other kinds of relaxation therapy.

Arthritis Relief at Your Fingertips gives the reader hands-on, practical suggestions for many types and stages of arthritic and rheumatic conditions. Results obtained may vary with the condition, its severity, and other factors. Well-established or advanced arthritic diseases may respond less well than earlier, mild cases. On the other hand, easily reversible conditions such as fibromyalgia, fibrositis, and myofascial syndrome may go into complete remission with the help of acupressure treatments.

Acupressure offers relief with no risk and at the same time is inexpensive and easily integrated into one's life. Michael Gach's arthritis exercises are easy to learn and easy to do. I strongly recommend this book to sufferers of arthritis or related soft tissue rheumatic disorders who are not satisfied living with chronic pain.

Murray C. Sokoloff, M.D.
Rheumatologist
Assistant Clinical Professor of Medicine,
Stanford University Medical Center

FOREWORD II

Prince Charles and an impressive number of respected British physicians use the term "complementary medicine" to refer to what Americans call "alternative medicine." Various natural healing modalities, which are becoming exceedingly popular in Great Britain and Europe, are no longer simply an alternative to conventional medicine; they are becoming an integral part of good medical care.

A growing number of physicians throughout the world are beginning to utilize nutrition, homeopathic medicine, acupuncture, biofeedback, botanical medicine, and various body therapies as part of this new development. This movement has been matched by the growing participation of the general public in a host of self-care methods. We are becoming conscious of the innate self-healing mechanisms that we as humans all share, departing from the mentality of being passive participants in our own health care and well-being.

Acupressure is a good example of a natural therapy that people can easily utilize at home with positive and beneficial results. Developed over thousands of years, acupressure is a nontoxic, non-invasive, sophisticated system to stimulate the healing process. In the same way that people of all cultures instinctively touch, rub, or press different parts of the body to relieve pain or discomfort, most of us have practiced and received the benefits of acupressure without even knowing it.

Once you learn basic acupressure techniques, you can do it anywhere, any time. The benefits are as close as your own fingertips. In my own life, it has relieved many an ache and pain. I have used it to help release pent-up emotions, to reduce day-to-day stress, and even to improve the quality of my skin and face.

Michael Reed Gach's *Arthritis Relief at Your Fingertips* is a no-nonsense guide to learning the practical applications of acupressure. This book is not only of value to those people with arthritis, but to anyone who feels stiffness, tension, or poor circulation in any part of their body.

As we approach the twenty-first century, acupressure and other healing methods will become a key part of our daily life. We may even wonder how we ever did without it.

Lindsay Wagner
Actress

ACKNOWLEDGMENTS

I want to thank entertainer Mary Martin for inspiring me to develop this Arthritis Relief Program. After I used acupressure to make her arthritic hands feel better, she jokingly asked me to go home with her; then, in a much more serious tone, Mary asked me to show her how to relieve arthritis using acupressure techniques, gentle stretching, and self-massage. My answer to that question eventually developed into this book.

I am indebted to Dana Ullman and Jim Spira for their support and professional resources; Frank Nuessle for his spiritual dedication and backing and to his Enhanced Media Group for producing high quality arthritis relief video and audio tapes; and Jack Howell for his guidance in the book trade.

I am grateful for my friendship with Scott Catamus and Katherine Ridall who introduced me to Cathy Hemming. She had the golden key that opened the doors at Warner Books. Joann Davis, Warner's senior editor, deserves to be acknowledged for reorganizing the manuscript into a comprehensive whole. I am grateful for the opportunity that Warner Books gave me to produce the layout, design, and graphics of this book.

I would like to acknowledge Elizabeth Rosner for her help in researching and writing introductions to sections and for editing the manuscript several times. I want to thank Lyn Lamb, who typed and retyped the manuscript through its many drafts; Sally Zahner who did an outstanding job of proofreading; Judith Jang, for her graphic design consultation and artistic direction; and Ann Marie Ericksen, who helped me paste up the manuscript. I especially want to thank Patricia Reilly for her supportive input, which helped me through the last draft; Mary Sanichas, whose desktop publishing talents created the inner mechanicals of the book; Joan Carol whose great artistic talents created the anatomical drawings; and David Lehrer for his expertise in shooting the photographs.

I would also like to express my appreciation to Lorraine Barret, Molly Beck, Gene Poferl, Fran Leftwich, Terry Calas, Herb Jorgensen, and Maureen Glew who modeled in the photographs.

I am deeply grateful for the loyal and dedicated teachers and staff at the Acupressure Institute. Without the support of Kathy Moring, who single-handedly manages the administrative demands at the Institute, I would never have had the time even to pick up a pen — let alone fly to Maui. I want to thank Mary Joan Dietrich who gave me her home for a month in Maui, where I had a healthy place to swim and write this book.

I want to thank Alice Hiatt, R.N.; Joey Carter, C.A.; Connie Cronin, C.A.; Janet Oliver, C.A.; Joseph Helms, M.D.; Charles May, M.D.; Dean Ornish, M.D.; Kenneth J. Zubrick, M.D.; Jonathan Shore, M.D.; and Murray Sokoloff, M.D., for reviewing the manuscript and giving me their medical advice.

Finally, I wish to acknowledge my parents for all the love, trust, and support they have given me to persevere in my goals and aspirations.

PREFACE

Arthritis affects more than 35 million Americans: it is the nation's number one crippling disease. If you are among the afflicted, your symptoms may be occasional or frequent, and you may suffer from swelling in one or more joints, recurring pain or tenderness in any joint, early morning stiffness, or an inability to move a joint normally. Whether your symptoms are mild or severe, they undoubtedly have a direct effect on your daily life. Perhaps you've been counseled about "learning to live with arthritis." But there is far more you can do to relieve your pain, increase your range of motion, and both relax and strengthen your muscles. As a recent handbook advises:

> One of the most important things you can do to help your arthritis is to exercise, if you do it right. Unfortunately, many people with arthritis think exercise is harmful. Others become discouraged because progress is slow or their exercises are painful. Maintaining a proper balance between rest and exercise, and exercising properly, are keys to a successful arthritis exercise program.[1]

In this book, you will learn techniques for relaxing muscles — techniques designed to decrease joint inflammation and relieve pain. Medical research tells us that movement is necessary for the proper nourishment of joint cartilage. When properly performed, these exercises and acupressure techniques enable the synovial fluid, which lubricates the joint, to carry the needed nutrients to the joints and to remove waste products.

If you don't use a muscle or joint, you'll lose strength and mobility, and, thus, function. If you've already lost function, remember it didn't happen in a day; it will take more than a day to regain it, especially if your arthritis is severe or if joint limitations have existed for a long time. By regularly practicing the self-help routines in this book, you will not only relieve your pain temporarily, but you will prevent an increase in symptoms and improve your overall well-being.

The acupressure massage techniques in this book are ideal for the treatment of arthritic conditions. As Paul Davidson, M.D. advises:

> Properly done, massage has many beneficial effects. It causes the muscles to relax and their nutrition to improve owing to an increase in blood flow. Muscles, scar tissue, and tendons are stretched, improving motion. The general overall effect on the body is one of sedation (a good alternative to drugs).

[1] Kate Korig and James F. Fries, *The Arthritis Helpbook*, Addison-Wesley, 1980.

People who have experienced <u>shiatsu</u>
[a form of acupressure massage] gen-
erally agree that although not initially
as soothing as as Swedish massage,
this form often provides excellent tem-
porary relief of localized pains and
good muscle relaxation.[2]

[2] Paul Davidson, M.D., *Are You Sure It's Arthritis?*,
Macmillan, 1985, p. 170.

A WORD TO THE WISE

This book is designed as a resource for people who suffer from arthritis and rheumatism. The exercises and procedures in this book are not a cure for arthritis, but are helpful for increasing circulation, and improving muscular flexibility and endurance. Gentle daily stretching along with acupressure point stimulation has been found effective for relieving tension and stiffness, as well as alleviating some of the aches and pains associated with arthritis and rheumatism.

If you're on medication, after months of regularly practicing the daily routines in this book, you may find that due to an increase in circulation you don't need as much medication as originally prescribed. If practicing these exercises seems to affect your metabolism, medication, and/or pain, be sure to consult your physician before changing the regimen that has been prescribed.

Note: If you have rheumatoid arthritis, consider these self-help techniques an important part of your treatment. Use the Arthritis Relief methods in this book, along with an overall medical treatment program advised by your doctor, a carefully planned mixture of activity and deep relaxation, and regular physical therapy treatments.

GUIDELINES FOR PRACTICING
ARTHRITIS RELIEF

For best results, once you're familiar with the Arthritis Relief techniques outlined in this book, I suggest you *spend about twenty minutes two or three times a day*, on the self-help techniques here. I recommend that you practice the routines in at least two of these chapters, once a day:

- " **The 12 Arthritis Relief Points**" (Chapter IV)
- " **Daily Routines**" (choose one routine) (Chapter V)
- " **Pain Relief for Specific Areas**" (choose one section based on where you arthritis is located) (Chapter VI)

In fact, the effectiveness of this Arthritis Relief program is contingent upon regular practice of these self-help techniques. Be prepared to spend some extra time, initially, as you learn the points and routines, and work slowly on building up your endurance. Also, make every effort to follow the basic dietary guidelines recommended here.

I have found that it usually takes about six months of daily practice for most people to obtain substantial relief from their arthritic pains. Regardless of exactly how long it takes you to achieve control over your arthritis, the gratifying results can be maintained only by continued practice of these same techniques throughout your life.

The support of a professional acupressure practitioner can make your healing process faster and more dramatic. Without outside help, you need to have a high level of faith and perseverance to work through the more difficult stages of your arthritic pain. The road of self-treatment is long, but if you progress daily in practicing the arthritis relief techniques, you can relieve your aches and pains naturally, without relying on drugs that can have irritating side effects.

During the past ten years, I have seen hundreds of people successfully relieve and manage their aches and pains simply by taking the basic training program at the Acupressure Institute. The consistent support of receiving acupressure both in and out of classes has helped many people not only to learn this healing art but has enabled them to regain a strong sense of health and well-being.

THE DEVELOPMENT OF
THE ARTHRITIS RELIEF PROGRAM

I am often asked how I developed this program. After years of studying and practicing many different holistic health modalities, I created this self-care system by integrating a number of natural therapeutic techniques designed to relieve stress and pain. My empirical research over the past 15 years has shown that increased effectiveness for relieving arthritic pain results from combining the key acupressure points with specific posture, movement, and breathing techniques.

My experience with arthritis sufferers has included both personal clients and many of the 60,000 people I have reached through classes and presentations. I have found — and my work with clients has proven — that gently holding the key acupressure points close to and directly on the arthritic sites significantly relieves the pain. The large number of people (including Mary Martin) who expressed interest in learning self-acupressure for their arthritis, along with my consistent success in relieving all kinds of aches and pains, encouraged me to write this book.

In 1976 I founded the Acupressure Institute in Berkeley, California, inspired by tremendous public interest in this hands-on healing art. Now in its second decade, the Institute has become one of the most comprehensive acupressure training centers in America, with people from all parts of the world coming to study with me, my senior instructors, and my staff.

In 1978 I originated Acu-Yoga, a self-acupressure stress management system that not only relieves aches and pains, but enables people to develop renewed, vibrant health.[3]

In the public arena, Mary Martin was the first person to ask me about how to use acupressure to relieve arthritis. When she pointed out the various arthritic joints on her hands, I showed her how to hold points that would relieve her pain. Mary insisted that I present self-care methods to enable people with arthritis to be self-reliant. After I demonstrated how to relieve shoulder and neck tension (as illustrated in this book), Mary tried it out for herself and exclaimed, "This is the first time my neck has felt well in years!"

I have found two major levels of relief, namely short and long-term results. First, most people experience some initial relief fairly immediately, of course, if they are doing these techniques properly. Most of the people I have worked with who have chronic, long-term arthritis have waves of both progress and setbacks. Do not expect an immediate cure. From my clinical experience, I have found that people who have had a history of arthritis must consistently practice *Arthritis Relief at Your Fingertips* to achieve the long-term benefits. It definitely takes work to accomplish the goals of pain relief and prevention naturally, without drugs. The best results come from steady practice of a combined program of easy-to-do stretching exercises and self-acupressure three times a day.

My positive experiences working with arthritis sufferers motivated me to conduct a preliminary study using the techniques in this book. This private research, using a group of 40 arthritis patients, is the focus of my Ph.D. thesis at

---

[3] *Note:* Michael Reed Gach's first book appeared several years later: *Acu-Yoga: Self-Help Techniques*, Japan Publications, distributed by Harper & Row, 1981.

Columbia Pacific University. With the guidance of my mentor, Jonathan Shore, M.D., we have been able to show that the techniques in this book were indeed helpful to well over a majority of the arthritic population tested. I hope that additional research will be conducted in the near future to further verify the benefits of these Arthritis Relief techniques.

Michael Reed Gach
April 1988

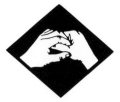

CHAPTER I

ACUPRESSURE FOR RELIEVING ARTHRITIS

ACUPRESSURE FOR RELIEVING ARTHRITIS

ACUPRESSURE HEALTH CARE

As a healing art, acupressure is as old as instinct itself — the spontaneous holding of a place on the body that is aching, wounded, or tense. The impulse that makes one double over and press one's stomach in response to abdominal cramps is an example of the instinctive practice of acupressure; it may well be the most ancient form of physical therapy.

More than five thousand years ago, the Chinese discovered certain points on the body which — when pressed, punctured, or heated — had a beneficial effect at the painful site and on certain ailments. Gradually, through trial-and-error and the sharing of experience, more and more points were discovered that were found not only to alleviate pain but also to influence the functioning of certain internal organs. Now it has been proven scientifically that these points have a lower skin resistance, that is, they transmit a greater current of human energy that is necessary for staying healthy.

Acupressure has much in common with acupuncture, a method of traditional Chinese medicine in which fine needles are inserted into the body. Acupuncture and acupressure use the same points to promote healing through the release of tension and the increase of blood circulation. The fundamental distinction lies in the needles used in acupuncture and the gentle but firm pressure of hands (and feet in some techniques) used in acupressure. Although the Chinese have developed more "technological" methods for stimulating points with needles and electricity, the older of the two modalities — acupressure — continues to be more effective in the relief of tension-related ailments, in self-treatment, and in preventive health care. A series of acupressure sessions or acupuncture treatments has been found especially helpful for relieving rheumatism[4] and arthritic pain.[5, 6]

Pressure acupuncture (commonly known as acupressure) can help the sufferer of arthritis whether traumatic, tendonitis as well as any ligamentous injury that is not severe enough to require surgery.[7]

---

[4] Katsusuke Serizawa, M.D., *Tsubo*, Japan Publications, 1976, pp. 142 and 143.

[5] Medicine & Health Publishing Co., *The Treatment of 100 Common Diseases by New Acupuncture*, 1984, pp. 22 and 23.

[6] Shanghai College of Traditional Medicine, *Acupuncture: A Comprehensive Text*, Eastland Press, 1981, pp. 606 and 607.

[7] Kenyon Keith, M.D., Pressure Points, *Do It Yourself Acupuncture Without Needles*, Arco Publishing Company Inc., 1977, p. 15.

Acupressure techniques are based on the principle that illness can be the result of stressors (internalized tensions) challenging the body's natural balancing mechanisms beyond their limits. The resulting pain, tensions, and constrictions inhibit the body's ability to effectively cope with the disrupting condition. In order to relieve pain, relax muscular tension, and balance the vital life forces of the body, acupressure concentrates on a system of points (around which muscular tension tends to accumulate) and meridians (which are the pathways along which the bio-electrical energy flows from point to point).

Consistent with the emphasis of traditional Chinese health care on the prevention of illness, acupressure treats symptoms as an expression of the condition of the person as a whole. Thus acupressure treatments focus not only on relieving pain and discomfort, but also on responding to tensions and toxins in the body before they develop into illnesses, that is, before the constrictions and toxins have caused damage to the internal organs.

ARTHRITIS PAIN RELIEF

There are special points on the body that, when held properly, relieve pain in the joints as well as muscular aches and pains. These are the same points that are used in acupuncture, but instead of using needles, you can stimulate these highly potent spots on the body through simple finger pressure.

Arthritis, which literally means "joint inflammation," tends to concentrate around these acupressure points. When the joints become chronically inflamed — the classic signs of arthritis — the build-up of pressure causes various types of nagging pain. Acupressure helps to relieve the joint pain by relaxing the muscles, enabling blood to flow freely. This relaxes the muscles surrounding the joints, and with daily practice of acupressure the arthritic pain can be greatly reduced.

An increase in circulation also brings more oxygen and other nutrients to affected areas. And when our blood and energy are circulating properly, we experience not only a natural decrease of pain, but a greater sense of aliveness and well-being. In Chinese medicine, acupressure points are considered gateways for "chi," the human electrical energy that runs throughout the body. This energy functions to regulate all systems of the body, and its unrestricted flow is the key to pain relief.

I helped treat [with Chinese massage] more than one hundred patients over two months... Every patient who entered that clinic [in China] felt dramatically relieved after thirty to sixty minutes of massage. There were no exceptions...

It was unmistakably clear... that massage, when applied appropriately, made every patient markedly more comfortable and more relaxed, within minutes and without drugs.[8]

---

[8] David Eisenberg, M.D., *Encounters With Qi*, Penguin, 1985, p. 113.

HOW ACUPRESSURE WORKS

Several theories exist to explain how acupressure relieves pain. One explanation is the "pain gateway" theory, which suggests that the transmission of pain impulses can be altered by inhibiting the pain signals sent to the brain. Acupressure (and acupuncture needles) produce a mild, fairly painless stimulation which closes the "gates" of the pain signalling system; thus, painful sensations cannot pass through the spinal cord to the brain.[9]

A second theory posits that when you hold acupressure points for long periods of time (more than one minute), the body releases neuro-chemicals called endorphins. The mechanism of endorphins is similar to morphine; both mitigate pain and encourage relaxation. However, endorphins are manufactured naturally by the body to promote healing. Acupressure stimulates this organic process, enabling the body to produce its own "natural painkillers."

> *Both generalized total body massage and focal massage are very useful techniques in controlling pain. Generalized massage helps create a feeling of relaxation and comfort, and is often very useful in helping patients to gain increasing mobility of joints.*[10]

ABOUT STRESS

Naturally, the amount of stress and tension in your life can affect your pain. All of the lifestyle factors that affect your health and well-being — e.g., how you handle tension, your posture, diet, the amount of exercise you get, etc. — also influence your arthritic condition. Like a computer, the human body picks up and stores biological information inside it. Emotional stress and repressed feelings, for instance, become physically ingrained in the muscles. These tensions often contribute to cause weaknesses in your general constitution, resulting in aggravated joints and pain. Part of our program will address the issue of reducing overall stress.

HOW TO FIND THE POINTS

Of the hundreds of acupressure points on the body, most either lie underneath major muscle groups or follow the bone structure, residing in the joints or in the hollows of bone. Each point can be found in relation to physical anatomical landmarks, such as the belly button, a specific muscle, or the crease behind the knee. As you read through the chapters of this book, you will be able to use your fingertips to feel for the major landmarks illustrated and described to locate the appropriate point.

In order to find an acupressure point with your hands, concentrate on feeling for a muscular cord or a hollow in the bone structure. Feel for a slight indentation or depression between the tendons and muscles at each point. Once you

[9] Leng T. Tan, Margaret Y. C. Tan, and Ilsa Veith, *Acupuncture Therapy — Current Chinese Practice,* Temple University, 1973.

[10] Normal Shealey, M.D., *The Pain Game,* Celestial Arts, 1976, p. 95.

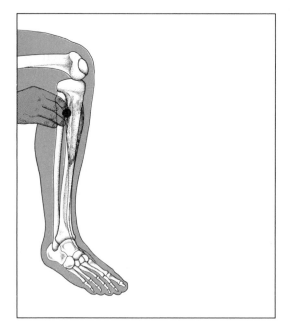

have found a muscular cord, press directly on it; or if you feel a bony hollow, slowly press directly into it at a 90-degree angle from the surface of the skin.

ACUPRESSURE POINT NUMBERING SYSTEM

In this book, we will be identifying the twelve most important acupressure points for the prevention and relief of arthritic pain. Additional acupressure points will be presented as well; however, do not be concerned about the complex numbering system assigned to these points. References such as "Sp 9" or "St 36" relate to the traditional acupuncture/ acupressure point system, and are provided for the benefit of acupressure and acupuncture professionals. *You do not need to know or remember any of these numbers to practice the Arthritis Relief Program.*

HOW TO PRESS THE POINTS

Although each point will feel somewhat different from the others, often the point is indicated by some degree of soreness upon pressure. If there is extreme (or increasing) sensitivity or pain, gradually decrease the pressure until a balance is achieved between pain and pleasure. It is important to use prolonged finger pressure directly at the site of your arthritic pain: a gradual, steady, penetrating pressure for three to five minutes is ideal. You should find that the initial pain you feel from the finger pressure is simultaneously relieving the arthritic pain. When you hold the point long enough, using the middle finger (with your index and ring fingers on either side for support), the pain will diminish, indicating that the acupressure is working.[11]

After repeated sessions with different depths of pressure, you will begin to feel a pulse at the arthritic pain sites; this is a good sign — it means increased circulation. Try to pay attention to the type of pulse you feel. If it's very light and faint, hold the point even longer until you feel the pulse grow fuller and deeper. If the pulse is throbbing, continue to hold the point until you feel the pulse become more regular.

---

[11] The middle finger is the longest and strongest of your fingers. Normally the thumb is strong too, but it lacks sensitivity. If your hand is weak or painful when you apply finger pressure, it is perfectly acceptable to use the knuckles of your fist or other tools such as an avocado pit, golf ball, or a pencil eraser.

Although you may be tempted to massage or rub the entire arthritic area, it's best to hold the point steadily with direct finger pressure. This is the most effective way to relieve your pain. If your hand gets tired, slowly withdraw pressure from the point, gently shake out your hand, and take a few deep breaths. When you're ready, go back to the point and gradually apply pressure until you reach the depth where it "hurts good." Again, hold directly on the painful site (which often moves, so stay with it), until you feel a clear, regular pulse or until the arthritic pain diminishes.

The "rule of thumb" for touching the points is to apply pressure at a 90-degree angle (diagonally) to the surface of the skin. It is important to remember always to apply your pressure gradually. The better your ability to concentrate on pressing your hand or fingers slowly on the point, the more effective you will be. Make your hands strong and graceful in applying pressure gradually.

Another important principle is to use your body by leaning your weight into the point. This is very important, even if you are predominantly using your hand to grasp or squeeze the point. Gradually lean your weight toward the point as you apply pressure, and stay on the point as you take several long, slow, deep breaths. Hold each point for at least three minutes as you breathe deeply.

Remember to go into and come out of the acupressure points as slowly as possible. The gradual application and release of pressure allows the tissues to respond and promotes healing.

Every body and every area of the body will require a different amount of pressure. If it hurts a great deal when you apply pressure on a point or arthritic joint, then use touch instead of pressure. A very light touch, without any rubbing, can be very effective for relieving soreness, inflammation, and arthritic pain.

There are certain areas of the body that tend to be sensitive, such as the calves, face, and genital areas. Many people like deeper pressure in the areas of the back, buttocks, and neck. The right amount of pressure varies from person to person, depending upon the amount of exercise he or she gets. The more developed a person's muscles are, the more pressure you should apply.

HOW TO USE ACUPRESSURE TO RELIEVE PAIN

The Arthritis Relief points can easily be practiced while sitting in a comfortable chair, but for the very best results, press these points while lying down in a relaxed, comfortable position with your eyes closed. Hold the painful joints and nearby acupressure points (illustrated throughout the book) for at least three minutes, breathing deeply into your abdomen; the breathing helps the points release and enables healing energy to circulate into your arthritic joints and throughout your whole body. Relaxation and a feeling of well-being will emerge the more you practice self-acupressure as a daily routine.

One way to easily find the exact location of an acupressure point is to firmly massage the area where you have pain. Inflammation, tension, or pain often centers on these points. After you find the pressure point that seems most directly connected to your pain, simply hold your fingers there for a few minutes without moving. Then feel for a tight muscular band, cord, knot, or inflamed tissue, and again hold directly on it for a few minutes without moving your fingers. Always go into the points very slowly and release your pressure gradually, ending with a steady, light touch.

A spot that is painful should be held gently without any movement for at least three minutes. Soreness upon pressure indicates some degree of blockage in the circulation surrounding the point. Do not press quickly or firmly on any sore area.[12] Several minutes of finger pressure applied very gradually on your arthritic pain spots helps to close the gates of your pain.

Sometimes when you are holding a point, it will cause a pain in another part of the body. This is known as "referred pain," which indicates that those areas are related. Note where these extra sore places are, and hold those spots as well. For increased effectiveness, remember to breathe deeply and allow yourself to completely relax with your eyes closed for a few minutes after practicing the arthritis relief methods.

Deep relaxation is the key to obtaining the maximum benefits from acupressure and other arthritis pain relief exercises. It is how you treat yourself through deep relaxation after doing these techniques that truly completes the healing process. For the very best results, encourage yourself to take a little nap after practicing your arthritis pain relief routine. This deep sleep, even if it's just for a few minutes, will help to heal, stabilize, and strengthen your joints.

---

[12] *Note:* If your arthritis flares up, in other words, if any area of your body becomes alarmingly inflamed, red, or very sore, give that part a day or two of rest.

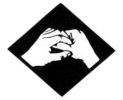

CHAPTER II
QUESTIONS
AND
ANSWERS

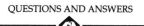

QUESTIONS AND ANSWERS

Before we get to the exercises, let me answer a few questions that I am commonly asked.

1. **What does acupressure do for arthritis?**
   The acupressure and stretching exercises in this book gently stimulate all parts of the body, relieving muscular tension and thereby increasing blood circulation. Western medicine is just beginning to recognize the importance of daily exercise, stress reduction activities, and the relationship between chronic muscular tension and many pain disorders.
   What is new to Western medicine is the idea that in traditional Chinese medicine stimulation of various trigger points on the body may help its organs and other parts. I suggest to my clients that they consult with their doctor for diagnosis and treatment. I make it perfectly clear that acupressure and the easy-to-do self-help techniques in this book can be an excellent adjunct but should not be considered a substitute for medical care.

2. **Will these techniques cure my arthritis?**
   No. However, they may substantially relieve your arthritis pain to help you feel better and more relaxed. Many people are discovering that gentle stretching and the use of massage are important means of relieving discomfort.

3. **What are the techniques in this book based on?**
   Arthritis Relief At Your Fingertips is based on points and principles of traditional Chinese medicine that emphasize preventing illness, dealing with underlying causes in depth, and treating the whole person. Each exercise naturally stimulates a series of key acupressure points.

4. **How long does it take to realize the benefits of your program?**
   A maximum of fifteen minutes a session, two or three times a day, is all you need. I have designed three basic daily stretch routines to choose from. The Acupressure Daily Stretch Routine, a morning wake-up set of self-massage techniques, takes fifteen minutes. The Midday Refresher series and the Evening Relaxation routine each take ten minutes. At first, the routines will take longer since you are not accustomed to the exercises. As you get to know the progression, they should go smoothly

and more quickly.

Most people feel some kind of partial relief after just a few times practicing these techniques. It usually takes six months of working on yourself two or three times daily to obtain substantial results. Once you reach this stage, it is important to do at least fifteen minutes of your favorite acupressure points and exercises twice a day to maintain your health and prevent further relapses.

5. **Are there basic rules to follow when practicing these techniques?**
Make your movements slow, graceful, and rhythmic. Be aware of your body and your posture. Keep a calm and alert presence of mind. Allow yourself to let go of your other involvements and responsibilities while you consciously practice these exercises. The therapeutic benefits increase when your mind and body work together.

Choose to practice the exercises that you enjoy. Do those that suit your physical condition and personal comfort. Be sure not to overdo any one particular exercise. Very gradually increase the amount of time you practice these techniques to develop stamina. If you exercise longer than a few minutes, allow yourself to completely relax with your eyes closed for a few minutes at the end. Deep relaxation will enhance the benefits.

6. **Do I need to believe in Eastern medicine and acupuncture to realize the benefits?**
No, of course not. Just try out the routines and notice for yourself what effects they produce.

7. **Where should these techniques be practiced?**
You can do them anywhere — at home, at the office, or even while waiting for a bus. However, some of the techniques are more appropriately practiced in private, like the "Tarzan Chest Pound." Other self-massage techniques, like the hand massage, neck rub, etc., can easily be done in all sorts of situations.

8. **What should I wear?**
You can do these exercises fully dressed, though lighter clothing is preferable. It is not necessary to wear "exercise" clothes. Many people like to wear a comfortable pair of shorts and a T-shirt.

9. **When is it preferable to do the Arthritis Relief techniques?**
You can do these routines anytime. For convenience, I have provided daily routines for the morning, midday, and evening. The morning routine is generally done soon after you wake up, but the routine can be practiced at any time of day. The midday series could be done at anytime, even a number of times during a hectic day. The evening routine is a good relaxation program to do before bed, but it could also be done at any time. Along with these

daily routines, also be sure to practice the techniques from other chapters in this book that cover specific areas where you have pain or tension. For instance, if you have arthritis in your fingers, try out the self-help techniques in the chapter on hands. Practice a few of your favorite exercises for your specific area of pain either after doing one of the daily routines or as a special individualized set of exercises for relieving your arthritis.

10. **Is it important to follow the routines exactly?**
No, but I recommend that at first you follow the routines as instructed. After you have thoroughly learned them, you can adapt the techniques to your own needs and preferences.

11. **If I have a neck injury, should I avoid these exercises?**
No, not necessarily. After an accident or injury, many muscles constrict. Acupressure can help loosen your tense muscles and improve circulation. If your neck is sensitive, be careful and do the routine gently. I suggest that you always check with your physician first.

12. **Should some of the routines hurt?**
The idea is not to cause pain. If something hurts, I suggest that you progress easily and gently. However, sometimes you will find areas of your body that are tense or highly sensitive, like your shoulders and neck. By pressing or gently touching, you help release some of the tension and bring relief.

13. **Can people who are ill or bedridden use these Arthritis Relief exercises?**
Yes. You do not have to be in the best of health to do these exercises, although I again suggest that you consult your doctor before adding my exercises to your daily routine.

14. **What age groups can practice these pain relief methods?**
These self-help techniques can be used by everyone, young and old alike. Once you are familiar with the routines, they become fun and easy. You can do them with your family. I have found that children love to do these exercises together with their parents or grandparents.

15. **Are these methods safe?**
As long as you use common sense. Always begin slowly and gently. As you practice, be aware of how your body feels. If you have any questions, I suggest that you consult your physician just as you would before beginning any exercise program.

16. **Do these methods take the place of exercise?**
No. Stretching and self-acupressure should not be confused with exercise, especially aerobic exercise, but you certainly can do them along with an exercise program if your physician does not object. And these exercises

can, of course, be done by themselves.

17. How can I incorporate these routines into my exercise program?

You might add some of the routines to your existing program, both at the beginning and at the end. After taking a brisk walk, for example, you might do a few leg exercises from the Acupressure Daily Stretch Routine to increase circulation and benefit the leg muscles. Or you might want to practice the evening relaxation techniques to calm and balance your whole body.

18. Can I do these self-help techniques to music?

You can if you want to. All types of music can be used to complement these Arthritis Relief self-treatments, from classical to more lively music. The evening routine is designed for relaxation, so if you do want to use music, it would be best to use the kind that helps you relax.

19. Can I use these methods on another person?

Most of these techniques are designed for self-application. However, some of the routines can certainly be done on a friend. The hands and feet techniques, for instance, can easily be done on oneself or someone else.

If you really want to learn how to do acupressure on others, study its many forms and styles: Acupressure Massage, Barefoot and Zen Shiatsu, Acu-Yoga, and Jin Shin Acupressure.

See page 219 of this book for more information about acupressure training.

20. Can I overdo these techniques?

Many good things can be overdone. I have deliberately made the routines short so that everyone can do them without strain. But if you really enjoy them, you may want to spend more time. Although twice or three times a day, totaling about an hour, is normally recommended, you can gradually and cautiously increase that to a maximum of two hours, keeping an awareness of the messages of your body as your guide.

21. Do I have to do the whole series or can I do just a few?

You can do only a few or all of them. You can create your own program. At first, however, I suggest you practice these Arthritis Relief exercises as presented.

22. Can pregnant women use these techniques?

First, consult your physician. During pregnancy, acupressure should be done gently, especially around the shoulders. If you are pregnant, I suggest that you avoid putting any pressure on your abdominal region and on the area between your thumb and index finger. These areas are forbidden to stimulate during pregnancy because they can trigger premature contractions in the uterus.

23. **What can I do to alleviate the worry I feel when I have pain? What factors often block a person's ability to help relieve his or her arthritis?**
When you catch yourself worrying or doubting, take some deep breaths and translate your concerns into reasons for loving yourself.

   In your search for a solution to relieving your arthritis, expectations often arise about obtaining a cure or immediate relief. Expectations tend to lead to disappointments, not to healing. In order to help yourself, you must listen to the messages of your body. That openness will enable you to know what your body needs, when and how much pressure to apply to specific joints, what your limitations are, how far to stretch, and when you need to relax. Instead of narrowly focusing on what you expect, you must be aware of your body's signals in order to take an active part in healing your arthritis naturally without drugs.

   We often want our pain to go away so badly that we expend energy worrying, complaining, or bitterly resenting the pain instead of focusing on where our constrictions are and which self-help techniques and acupressure points seem to directly affect those areas. In other words, try to replace your doubts, worries, and expectations (which only drain you of energy) with your willpower, your faith in the possibility of your healing, and trust in yourself to choose healthy activities and situations that give you greater energy, a sense of purpose and aliveness.

24. **In addition to the suggestions and techniques in this book, what can I do to further relieve my arthritic pain?**
Receiving several private acupressure massage or Jin Shin acupressure treatment sessions, and applying heat to the acupressure points (a method called moxabustion), done by an acupressure professional, can greatly relieve your arthritis. Plan to take a nap right after the treatment to maximize the benefits.

   To receive a directory of acupressure practitioners, send $3 to:

Acupressure Institute
1533 Shattuck Avenue
Berkeley, California 94709

   Also check your local health food store and spiritual bookstore for further references for acupressure practitioners and massage therapists. Acupuncturists, listed in the Yellow Pages, can also be of great help.

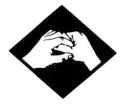

CHAPTER III

CAUSES
OF
ARTHRITIS

CAUSES OF ARTHRITIS

In this chapter, I would like to discuss the major causes and types of arthritis briefly, including an Eastern perspective. The background material here is not needed to practice the techniques that follow. So, if you are anxious to begin the Arthritis Relief exercises, feel free to skip this chapter and return to it later.

Arthritis can be caused by genetic family tendencies, streptococcus, chronic muscular tension, and other stress factors. This, along with a lack of movement and poor circulation, can eventually cause joint congestion, inflammation, and irritation.[13]

Diet may be another common contributing factor in some types of arthritis.[14] Many experts agree that it is helpful to cut back on a large consumption of red meat, hard cheese, salt, and sugar.[15] The more digestible your foods are, the less metabolic waste products there will be in the blood. It is best to substitute these foods with fresh vegetables (both cooked and raw), well-cooked whole grains (millet is the best), hot lemon water[16] (juice of one-half lemon mixed with a cup of hot water), and a moderate amount of fresh fruit in season.

Another very different cause of arthritis involves injury to the joints. This can occur from an accident such as a fall or severe sprain. When injuries do occur,

> ...an effective method of restoring the injured part to health is of great value. Pressure acupuncture can be of considerable assistance in achieving that end. For the person who is approaching or has reached middle age, proper exercise is important to health and well being. It becomes difficult to do this when one suffers from arthritis, bursitis, tendonitis, or a pulled muscle in a limb that is essential to carry out the exercise. There are a variety of names for such maladies, such as tennis elbow, pulled hamstring, charley horse or sacro-iliac trouble. Younger people may not suffer as much from arthritic ailments as their elders, but they are certainly susceptible to sprains and muscle pulls for which pressure acupuncture and acupressure massage can be a very useful treatment. And it can be used not only out on the playing fields but in the comfort of one's own living room while watching television.[17]

---

[13] Leonard Mervyn, *Rheumatism and Arthritis*, Thorons Science of Life Series, 1986, pp. 10 and 11.

[14] See the chapter on diet, foods, and recipes for more information.

[15] Naboru Muramoto, *Healing Ourselves*, Avon Publishers, 1973, p. 118.

[16] Elson Haas, M.D., *Staying Healthy with the Seasons*, Celestial Arts, 1981, p. 42.

[17] Keith Kenyon, M.D., *Pressure Points: Do-It-Yourself Acupuncture Without Needles*, Arco Publishing Company Inc., 1977, p. 15.

Arthritis can also develop as a result of overuse of one or more joints. Gymnasts are commonly prone, for example, to develop arthritis due to their strenuous activities. This type of arthritis requires joint protection and rest, along with the self-help techniques presented in this book.

FIVE MAIN TYPES OF ARTHRITIS

There are over a hundred types of arthritis, and it can be important to establish a correct diagnosis of the type of arthritis you have. I recommend a visit to a doctor who works with holistic health methods, such as exercise and nutrition, for an individual diagnosis, medical perspective, and advice.

In this chapter, we will first take a Western perspective and briefly discuss the five major types of arthritis.[18] Then we will explore the four major types according to traditional Chinese medicine.

1. **Osteoarthritis** is usually a mild condition involving the breakdown of cartilage and sometimes bone. Typically it affects the fingers, hips, knees, and spine. Regular exercise is extremely important in preventing and remedying existing osteoarthritic conditions.

2. **Rheumatoid Arthritis** is usually a much more serious condition that, in its most severe forms and without treatment, can result in joint deformity. Chronic inflammation can attack joints, skin, muscles, blood vessels, even the lungs and heart (in rare cases). It often affects many joints and causes whole-body illness as well as damage to joint tissues. Treatment of rheumatoid arthritis involves a balance between rest and activity, and a long-term conditioning program is best developed with the help of a physician.

3. **Systemic Lupus Erythematosis** most often affects women, and the condition appears in the skin, joints, and internal organs. Early diagnosis and treatment makes SLE more manageable.

4. **Ankylosing Spondylitis** is a condition affecting the spine, in which the bones of the spine fuse. It can also affect the shoulders, knees, ankles, eyes, heart, and lungs.

5. **Gout** is an acutely painful condition that currently affects about one million Americans, usually men. It results from a chemical defect that allows too much uric acid to build up in the body. During "gout attacks" uric acid forms crystals that become lodged in a joint, frequently the big toe, causing inflammation.

---

[18] For further information, read Dr. James Fries, *Arthritis, A Comprehensive Guide*, Addison-Wesley, 1979.

THE EASTERN PERSPECTIVE OF ARTHRITIS

According to traditional Chinese medicine, there are four main types of arthritis: wind, heat, cold, and damp. The wind type of arthritis, characterized by moving aches and pains, is often worsened by the wind. Heat arthritis is often reddish and noticeably inflamed. It may feel red and hot to the touch. Cold arthritis is characterized by swollen, painful joints that are sensitive to changes in humidity (e.g., rain, fog, or high relative humidity). Damp arthritis often aches during weather changes, especially when temperatures drop or storms are approaching.

It is important to note that these four types can combine in various ways. Before describing these combinations, it should be mentioned that wind is "the first evil" — that is, wind, which moves, can carry one of the other "evils" (heat, cold, damp) into the body with it. This is seen in the combination of wind and damp arthritis, a type of arthritis especially prevalent among the elderly. This syndrome is analagous to rheumatism in Western medicine. Its hallmark is coldness, swelling, and pain, responding to changes in the weather — cooler temperatures and/or signals of cold, damp weather. Many cultures note this syndrome in their folk beliefs by predicting weather changes according to changes in individuals' joints.

The other major combination is heat and damp. This combination is recognizable by red, swollen, and painful joints.

In Western medicine, this type of arthritis is called rheumatoid arthritis and is a very serious condition.

There are general and specialized acupressure points for dealing with these four types of arthritis. Point #1 is the

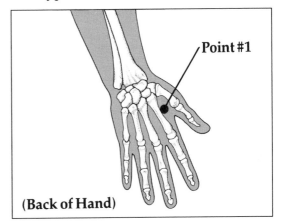

Point #1

(Back of Hand)

general, all-purpose point for relieving all four types. This anti-inflammatory point is located in the webbing between the thumb and index finger.

HEAT ARTHRITIS

The hot, reddish, inflamed type of arthritis can be helped by regularly stimulating the Sp 10 point.[19] This point is located on the inside of the thigh, three finger-widths above the top of your kneecap. The point will probably be tender upon pressure. Hold with a light but firm pressure until the soreness almost completely subsides.

WIND ARTHRITIS

This type of moving arthritic pain, which is sometimes accompanied by fever or chills, can be helped by Point #1 (between the thumb and index finger), Point #7, Point #9, Point #12, and GB 31.

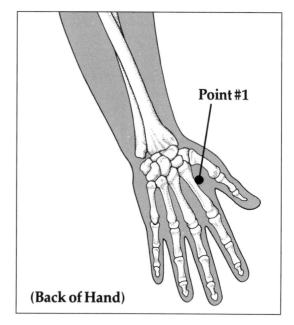

(Back of Hand)

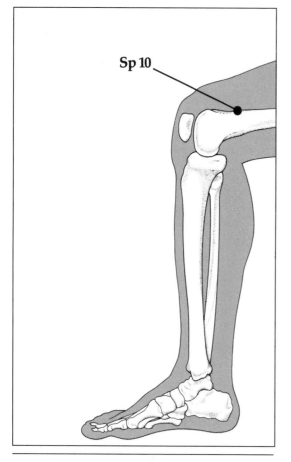

---

[19] These numbers refer to the acupuncture/acupressure point system of the body. Each point is on a pathway that is linked to and named after an internal organ.

Point #7 is located on the shoulder muscle just above the tip of the shoulder blade.

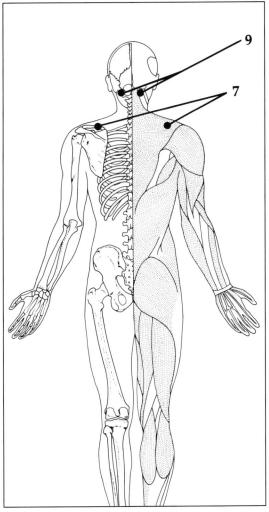

Point #9 is located underneath the base of the skull, halfway between the spinal column and the tip of the ear lobe. GB 31 is located on the extreme outside of the thigh between the knee and the hip bone. Your middle finger will be on GB 31 when you are standing with your

shoulders relaxed and your arms by your sides. Feel for the most sensitive spot on your thigh. Point #12 is located on the top of the foot between the bones that attach to the 4th and 5th toes. Slide your index finger one inch up from the webbing between the baby toe and the 4th toe. Feel for a sensitive spot, pressing between the bones just below where they juncture.

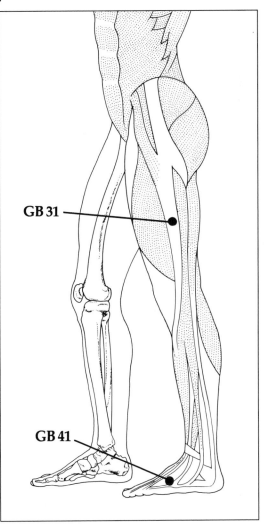

COLD AND DAMP ARTHRITIS

For the cold and damp types of arthritis, you will find that cold and movement will tend to aggravate the pain, whereas heat will help relieve the pain. Use the Stomach 36 point (St 36), located on the outer side of the lower leg, four finger-widths below the bottom of the kneecap.

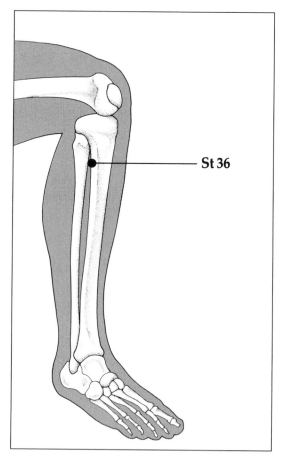

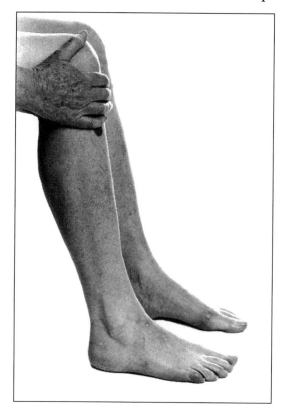

This point is underneath a muscle that will pop out when you bend your foot up and down. Stomach 36 helps relieve general muscle pains and is the most widely used point for revitalizing the entire body.

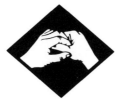

CHAPTER IV

THE
TWELVE
ARTHRITIS
RELIEF POINTS

THE TWELVE ARTHRITIS RELIEF POINTS

As we have noted, there are special acupressure points that strengthen specific joints and gradually rebalance the system and relieve arthritis and rheumatism. By stimulating these points daily with finger pressure and hot, wet compresses, you can improve your overall condition and manage your arthritis.

In this chapter, you will learn the twelve most important acupressure points for the prevention and relief of arthritic pain. Dr. Norman Shealy, M.D., director of the Pain Rehabilitation Center in Wisconsin, has acknowledged finding several of these points to be "most useful in the treatment of pain."[20]

In fact, if you count both the left and right sides of your body, you will find a total of twenty-four points, twelve on each side. This section numbers these points one through twelve and contains a description of the location, the proper way to apply finger pressure, as well as the benefits of these important Arthritis Relief points. At the end of this chapter, you will find specific instructions on how to press these points on yourself.

THE TWELVE ARTHRITIS RELIEF POINTS[21]	
Point 1 is LI 4	Point 7 is TW 15
Point 2 is Lu 10	Point 8 is B 10
Point 3 is TW 5	Point 9 is GB 20
Point 4 is LI 10	Point 10 is B 47
Point 5 is LI 11	Point 11 is St 36
Point 6 is SI 10	Point 12 is GB 41

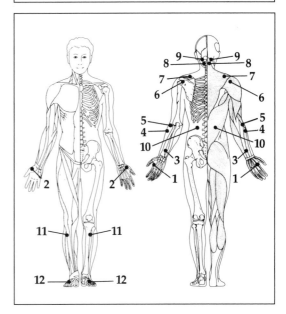

---

[20]Norman Shealy, M.D., *The Pain Game*, Celestial Arts, 1976, p. 95.

[21] These numbers refer to the acupuncture/acupressure point system of the body. Each point is on a pathway that is linked to and named after an internal organ. You do not need to know these numbers; they are primarily being listed here for professional reference purposes.

Point #1

Location: Point #1 is located at the highest spot of the muscle when the thumb and the index fingers are brought close together. Press in the webbing between the thumb and index finger, closer toward the bone that attaches to the index finger.

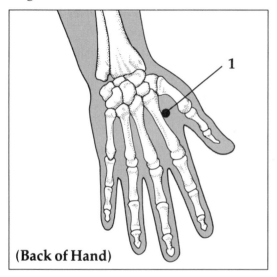

(Back of Hand)

Finger Application: Press into the muscle of the web (between the thumb and index fingers), angling the pressure towards the bone that connects with the index finger.
Benefits: This anti-inflammatory point has been used to relieve pain caused by arthritis in all parts of the body, particularly in the hands, wrists, elbows, and shoulders. It also has been used to relieve neck pain, migraine headaches, toothaches, constipation, and neuralgia.

Point #2

Location: Point #2 is located on the palm side of the hand in the center of the big mount at the base of the thumb.

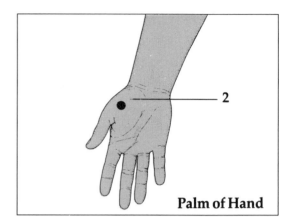

Palm of Hand

Finger Application: Apply firm pressure into the center of the fleshy pad where the thumb joins the palm of the hand.
Benefits: Relieves arthritis in the hand, coughing, swollen throat, upset stomach, anorexia, and alcohol abuse.

Point #3

Location: Point #3 is located by flexing your hand backward. The point is on the outside of the forearm, two finger-widths (approximately $1^{1/2}$ inches) from the wrist crease. Press in firmly between the forearm bones (radius and ulna).

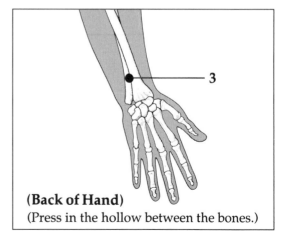

(Back of Hand)
(Press in the hollow between the bones.)

Finger Application: This point requires firm, prolonged pressure for best results. You can use either your thumbs or your fingers to stimulate the point, whichever is easier. To get firm pressure, wrap your hand around the wrist (1$^{1/2}$ inches from the crease) using both your fingers and thumb to clamp onto the outside and inside of your wrist. Hold this point firmly on each arm.

Benefits: Firm pressure on this point is also helpful for tightness or pain in the shoulders. As an important tonic, this point has been traditionally used to increase the body's resistance to colds and flu. Pressure on this point also balances and strengthens the whole body, especially improving the elasticity of the skin and the tone of the muscles.

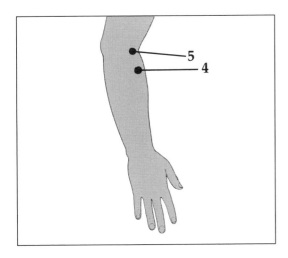

Point #4

Location: Point #4 is located by bending your arm to form a crease at the elbow joint. The point is located one inch toward your hand from the end of this crease, on a muscle.

Finger Application: When you flex your hand back and forth while holding this point with your other hand, you should feel the muscle pop out if you are on the correct spot. Apply pressure gradually into the center of that forearm muscle.

Benefits: This special anti-inflammatory acupressure point relieves arthritis anywhere in the upper portion of the body, especially in the hand, wrist, and elbow joints. When you feel tired or depressed, try pressing this forearm point. The point will often be sore, especially when you are feeling low or when your colon is congested. This is a great pain point to press for developing vitality in the upper portion of your body, as well as for relieving aching, tired muscles and joints. Try stimulating this point on both arms for one minute each when you get up in the morning.

This point is also traditionally used for muscular spasms in the arm and upper back, indigestion, a swollen or stiff neck, and poor circulation.

Point #5

Location: Point #5 is located in the elbow joint at the outer end of the crease where your arm bends.

Finger Application: Use your thumb to press deeply into the elbow joint with the arm partially flexed.

Benefits: Relieves joint inflammation, particularly in the elbow and shoulder joints. It also relieves constipation, skin problems, fever, high blood pressure, colds, flu, and depression, as well as general aches and pains.

Point #6

Location: Point #6 is located where the arm joins the back between the top of the shoulder bone and the back crease of the armpit.

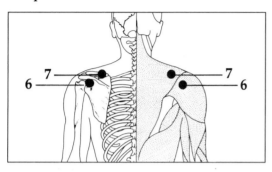

Finger Application: Press directly on the muscular cord in the shoulder joint, angling the pressure in toward the heart.
Benefits: Relieves arthritis, bursitis, and rheumatism, as well as releasing shoulder and upper back pain. Also, this point is traditionally used for hypertension, spontaneous aches and pains, insomnia, anxiety, nervousness, arm pain or numbness, and cold hands.

Point #7

Location: First find the spot on the top of the shoulder that is midway between the outside of the base of your neck and the outside of your shoulder. Point #7 is located one-half inch directly below this spot. Reach your right hand over your left shoulder, curving your fingers to hook onto the trapezius muscle on the top of your shoulders.
Finger Application: Press firmly on the shoulder muscles above the center of each shoulder blade.
Benefits: Relieves shoulder and neck

stiffness and pain, including rheumatism. This point also increases the resistance to colds and flu.

Point #8

Location: Point #8 is located on the upper portion of the neck, approximately one thumb's width outside the spine. Usually a lump of tension can be felt at this point.

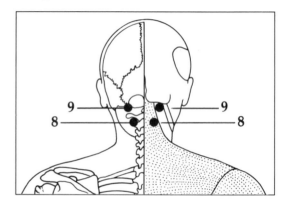

Finger Application: Grasp the back of your neck with one hand, using all your fingers on one side and the heel of your hand on the other side to firmly squeeze the ropy neck muscles.
Benefits: Key point for releasing stiffness, rigidity, and arthritic pain in the neck and back. Also strongly benefits the nervous system and is especially useful in times of stress and trauma.

Point #9

Location: Point #9 is located in the hollow below the base of the skull in between two muscles (the trapezius and the sternocleidomastoid). This point is often used to relieve pain and trauma after injuries.

Finger Application: Firm pressure underneath the hollow of the skull with the head tilted back. Hold both sides together.

Benefits: Relieves arthritic pains, headaches, hypertension, insomnia, back pain, eyestrain, stiff neck, irritability, nervousness, mental pressures, memory, neuromotor coordination problems, dizziness, and head colds.

Point #10

Location: Point #10 is located in the lower back (between the second and third vertebrae) a few inches out laterally from

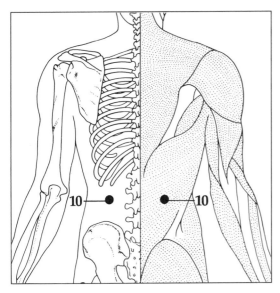

the spine at the level of the waist. This important lower back point can be found by pressing the outer edge of the large vertical muscles (that run alongside the spine) in toward the center of the vertebrae.

Finger Application: Use either your thumbs or the fingers of your hand to press the large ropelike muscles that run parallel to your spine, one side at a time or both sides at once. Another way to stimulate these points is to make fists and rub the lower back briskly with your knuckles.

Benefits: Relieves lower backaches, fatigue, reproductive problems, impotency, low sexual desire, vaginal discharge, and kidney and urinary problems.

Point #11

Location: Point #11 is located by measuring four finger-widths below your kneecap and one finger-width outside of your shinbone. If you are on the correct spot, a muscle should pop out as you flex your foot up and down.

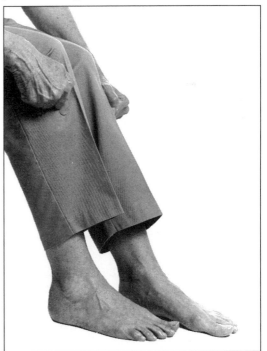

Point #11 *(Continued)*

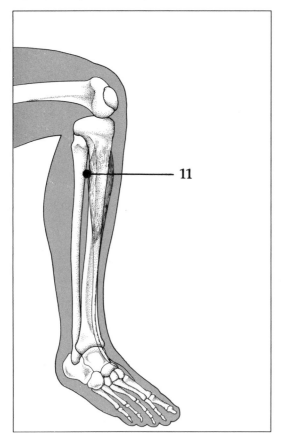

Finger Application: Using your own heel to briskly rub this point is one of the most effective methods for stimulating this point on yourself.

1. Place your right heel on Point #11 of your left leg and briskly rub it for one minute.
2. Reverse, and do the same on the other side.

Benefits: Counteracts arthritic pain in all parts of the body, especially pain in the knee joint. Firm pressure on this point immediately fortifies the body with

renewed energy. It helps to tone the major muscle groups, enabling one to have greater endurance. It is also among the most famous acupressure points known throughout China and Japan for alleviating sore, tired muscles and general fatigue.

Pressure on this point strengthens the whole body, tones the muscles, and aids digestion; it also relieves stomach disorders and fatigue.

Point #12

Location: Point #12 is located between the 4th and 5th metatarsal bones on the top of the foot.

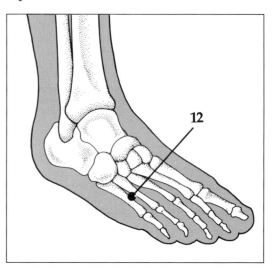

Finger Application: Place your fingertip between the 4th and 5th metatarsal bones, gliding your finger upward and pressing just below the juncture.

Benefits: Relieves hip and shoulder tension, roving pains, headaches, side aches, perspiration, rheumatism, excessive water retention, and sciatica.

SELF-HELP INSTRUCTIONS

The following step-by-step instructions will tell you how to stimulate each of the twelve Arthritis Relief points. Practice this self-acupressure massage routine on a daily basis.

1. Use the knuckles (illustrated) of your left fist to gradually apply pressure to Points 1-5 on your right arm for one minute each.

2. Use your left hand with your fingers

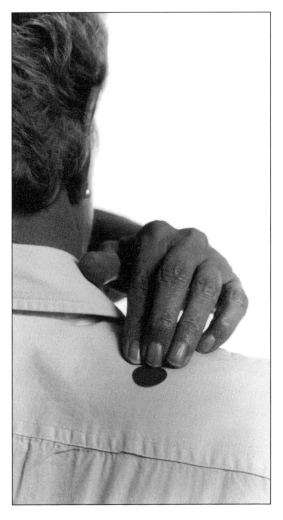

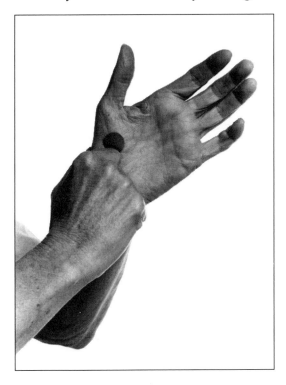

together and curved to hook onto Points 6 and 7 on the shoulders.

3. Repeat steps 1 and 2 (above) on the other arm, holding Points 1-5 with the knuckles on your fists and then Points 6 and 7 with your fingertips hooked onto your shoulders.

4. Use all of your fingertips to firmly hold Point 8 on both sides of your neck for one minute.

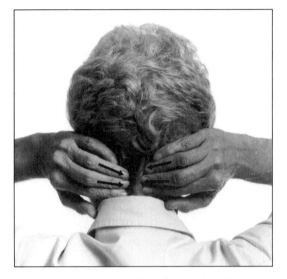

5. Then use your thumbs to firmly press Point 9 on both sides underneath the base of your skull for another minute.

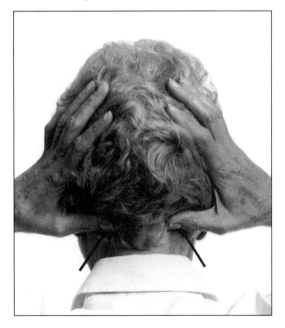

6. Place the back of your fists against Point 10 on both sides of your lower back. Briskly rub up (as far as you can comfortably reach) and down to your buttocks for one minute, creating warmth from the friction.

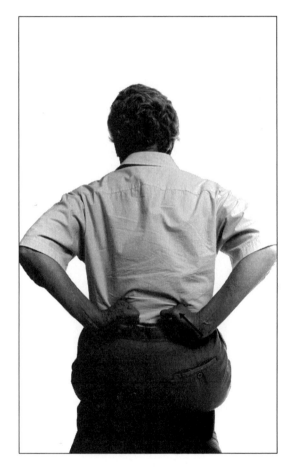

7. Next, place each of your fists on Point 11 on the outside of the both shinbones, below the knees. Briskly rub to stimulate the points for one minute. Try to spend extra effort and time to activate these vital points in order to increase the benefits.

8. Firmly press Point 12 on both sides with your fingers on the top of the foot for one minute.

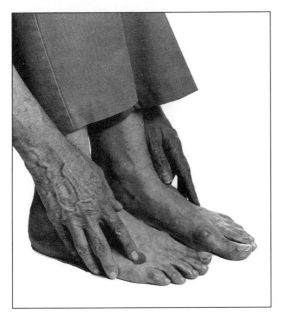

9. Congratulations, you have completed the acupressure massage routine that stimulates the most important anti-inflammatory points for relieving arthritis!

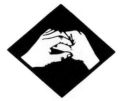

CHAPTER V

DAILY
ROUTINES

DAILY ROUTINES

ACUPRESSURE, STRETCHING AND BREATHING EXERCISES

This chapter will give you daily general exercise guidelines followed by simple instructions for practicing morning, afternoon, and evening routines; these easy, self-help exercises are designed to help you relieve and manage your arthritis. I highly recommend that you regularly practice the pain relief exercises in your daily life. You should do one of these routines every day, along with the more targeted self-help exercises illustrated in the next chapter entitled, "Pain Relief for Specific Areas."

GENERAL EXERCISE GUIDELINES

- **Regular daily practice** is the way to healthy, flexible joints. Start slowly and enjoy the movements. If you get interrupted while practicing, don't worry. Just continue where you left off, whenever it's convenient. After one month of regular daily practice, these exercises will become part of your everyday routine, something you miss if you don't do them. The results you experience will motivate you to continue.

- **Be consistent** about practicing the exercises you enjoy. Do the ones that

suit your physical condition and style. If an exercise "feels wrong" or increases your inflammation or pain, discontinue that technique. *Be sure not to overdo any one particular exercise.* Begin at a comfortable level for you, and gradually increase the intensity or the number of repetitions, working to develop stamina.

- **Make your movements and stretches slow**, graceful, and rhythmic. The daily routines in this chapter are holistically designed to work on all parts of the body, not just your painful arthritic areas. When practiced slowly and carefully, the arthritis pain relief exercises tone the muscles, gently stretch the tendons, and enable inflamed joints to heal. Keeping a steady rhythm in your movements increases the power and effectiveness of each exercise.

- **Be aware of your body posture** as you practice the routines. Proper posture is vital for correct deep breathing and helps the movements to be beneficial to the entire body.

- **Deep breathing** is the key to health as well as to a drug-free method for pain relief. Deep breathing is particularly important for an arthritic patient to practice, for it increases the amount of fully oxygenated red blood cells and helps fortify your body with the vital energy it needs to heal your inflamed joints. Tightness in your chest and lower back muscles constricts the ribs so they cannot work properly, causing you to breathe shallowly. When this muscle tension is released, the lungs can open to allow deep, full breathing.

You can strengthen your lungs and diaphragm through the practice of slow, deep breathing; increasing the volume of air you take in with each breath can help nourish and promote healing of painful, inflamed joints. Use the following steps as a guide for your deep breathing:

1. Breathe quietly for a minute, noticing how you breathe and letting yourself relax.

2. On an exhale, gently force all the air out of your lungs and diaphragm by pulling in your belly at the end of the exhalation.

3. Now inhale deeply. Your belly, having just been contracted, will naturally expand as you inhale. Visualize the breath being slowly gathered into your abdomen.

4. Continue, exhaling deeply by pulling in your belly, and inhaling deeply by letting your belly expand.

Many people spend a great deal of their time indoors, both at work and at home, and therefore get very little fresh air and exercise. Even if you live in an

area plagued by air pollution, it's better to get outside at least some time during the day to stretch, move, and breathe deeply.

- **Deep relaxation:** It is extremely important to give your muscles time to relax in between repetitions of each exercise. Completely relax immediately following the exercises to enhance the relief of arthritic pains and to allow increased circulation to remove waste products. If you exercise longer than a few minutes, allow yourself to completely relax on your back with your eyes closed for a few minutes. The combination of exercise and relaxation will increase both your enjoyment and the effectiveness of the pain relief program.

- **Warmth can help relax stiff muscles and joints**. You may want to apply heat prior to exercise to warm up the joints and relieve sore, stiff muscles. Take a hot bath or shower, or apply a hot water bottle or electric heating pad to the arthritic areas. Try to avoid becoming chilled, especially after you practice the exercises and self-acupressure.

- **Word of caution:** A joint should not be exercised when it is inflamed, or "hot" (swollen, red, tender to the touch). However, even those "hot" joints should be gently moved each day to maintain the joint's range of flexibility. It's best not to apply heat or deeply massage a "hot" joint;[22] instead, gently hold the inflamed area for a few minutes and apply a tofu plaster.[23]

- **If your arthritis flares up, see your doctor or physical therapist.** Your condition may be too advanced to completely eliminate all of your symptoms, but you can often prevent your arthritis from getting worse. When practiced daily, this set of stretches and self-acupressure massage will enable you to be more flexible and to feel much better.

- **Keep a calm and alert presence of mind.** Allow yourself to let go of your other involvements and responsibilities while you practice these exercises consciously. The therapeutic benefits increase when your mind and body work together.

MENTAL ATTITUDE

Your attitude about the arthritis pain relief exercises strongly affects your practice of them. A negative or judgmental attitude can strongly affect your participation and therefore the results. It is best simply to notice when your judgments and self-criticisms are getting in the way of fully practicing these routines. When you let go of expectations and negative judgments, you can focus more clearly on what you're doing and experience the benefits more directly. Focus on breathing deeply and keeping your attention on the here-and-now, with a positive, open attitude while you're practicing the exercises.

Many attitudes may surface while you are doing these exercises. For instance, you may get frustrated by your stiffness or pain and may not want to continue. Most likely you will have setbacks, depressions, upsets, or flare-ups that may make it difficult to continue practicing these exercises. You may have problems breathing deeply or focusing your attention on the daily routines. At this stage, it is as important for you to not only rely on your self-discipline, but also go to an acupressurist, massage therapist, counselor, or physical therapist for support and further guidance.

If you have a "flare-up" (which commonly occurs) and you think the exercises are aggravating the pain, take a day or two to rest and recuperate.

I am hopeful, however, that you will find a positive experience in which the exercises are fun, and it's a joy and challenge to move and stretch. You can use this positive attitude to further your progress.

Your will power is an important tool for improving the quality of your life. It enables you to realize your full potential, pursuing what you know is right, stretching both mind and body to live a deeper, fuller life. Cultivate this kind of attitude as you practice your exercises. And always put your heart into whatever you do.

---

[22] Kate Lorig and James F. Fries, *The Arthritis Helpbook*, Addison-Wesley, 1980.

[23] See the section on External Treatments on page 201 for instructions on how to make a tofu plaster.

LIFESTYLE AND PERSONALITY CONSIDERATIONS

As you prepare to fit these arthritis pain relief exercises into your daily routine, you will choose how and when according to your own lifestyle and personality. If you are the type of person who prefers discipline, then set up a schedule to practice regularly. Just as you manage to do other things you enjoy without making a big effort, you will be able to find the time and create the opportunity to practice these routines.

Try to keep your focus on the results that lie ahead. By the time you've been practicing regularly for a month, you will be likely to feel noticeable improvement. After a while, you won't need as much discipline to practice these arthritis relief routines because they will have become more enjoyable.

In addition to creating a structure that supports your practice of the daily arthritis relief exercises, you can also incorporate many of these same techniques into your current lifestyle. For example, at various times during the day, while watching TV or a movie, talking on the phone, reading, or even waiting in line, you can rotate your hands on your wrists, massage your shoulders or work on your hands by gently stretching and massaging your fingers. A simple movement such as reaching for a jar on a high shelf, for instance, can be an opportunity for you to practice self-help by reaching with your other arm too, and making it a complete stretching movement.

You may discover that the way you hold your body creates tension. You can then use the pressure points and stretches to relieve the pain and stiffness in your joints, and you can learn new ways of sitting and standing that don't cause tension. You can improve your posture and practice deep breathing while you hold points, and gently stretch tight, tired muscles.

Coming up with new ways of integrating these techniques into your daily life can be fun and most certainly can bring relief from stiffness and pain.

THE STAGES OF EXERCISE

Over a period of time practicing the exercises, you will probably go through a progression of stages. It can be frustrating at the beginning, when you first learn a new self-help technique. In this first stage, grasping the mechanical aspects of the exercise is often difficult.

In the second stage, however, the exercises become more refined movements, smooth and graceful. You may still have to concentrate on the mechanics of the exercise, but once you practice long enough, you will become more aware of your body and the dynamics of the movement.

The third stage of practicing these arthritis pain relief methods develops as you begin to master the exercises. At this point, the movements will become so familiar that you no longer have to concentrate on what you're doing. In this last stage, you experience your body truly flowing with the movements. Health, like any goal, must be earned by practice. Constant practice, at least twice daily, is the way to successful arthritic pain relief.

STARTING THE DAY OUT RIGHT

The following routines are a great way to fully wake up and enable you to be more limber throughout the day. Much of your morning stiffness will be relieved by doing these easy stretches and breathing exercises.

The first few exercises are designed to be done while still in bed, before you even arise. If you experience any sharp pains, stop immediately. Begin long, deep breathing to enable you to relax. Then proceed very slowly and with caution.

Whole Body Stretch
(Lying on your back)

1. *Stretch your arms* upward and over your head while taking a couple of slow, deep breaths.
2. *Stretch your legs* one at a time and then stretch both legs outward as you stretch your arms.
3. *Tighten your buttocks* a few times as you clench your fists with your hands at your sides. Then simply relax.

Good Morning Rotations
(Lying on your back)

1. *Rotate your feet* several times on your ankles as you take another couple of slow, deep breaths.
2. *Rotate your hands* on your wrists a few times.

3. *Roll your head* slowly and easily from side to side several times to help your neck become more relaxed.

Massage Your Face into a Smile

1. *Eyes:* Gently massage around your eyes, eyebrows, and then just above the bridge of your nose. To gently stretch the eye muscles: Close your eyes, take a deep breath through your nose (if possible), and roll your eyes up and backward. Take one more deep breath as you roll your eyes up to stretch them again.
2. *Temples:* Place your fingertips on your temples and slowly massage in a circular motion, keeping your eyes closed and your breathing full and deep.
3. *Cheekbones:* Press underneath (the whole length of) your cheekbones, using your fingertips on both sides of your face.
4. *Jaws:* Firmly massage your jaw muscles as you take a few long, deep breaths. Then let your jaws move from side to side, and again firmly massage to release any remaining jaw tension. Allow your mouth to be open to relax your jaw muscles.
5. *Ears:* Knead both of your ears until they feel warm and vibrant. Thoroughly massage all areas of your ears, covering inner as well as outer surfaces.
6. *The smile:* Take and deep breath and smile widely. Stretch your arms upward as you take another deep breath, and exaggerate your smile even more.

Make sure you take a hot bath or shower in the morning to warm up your joints. Then practice the following acupressure daily stretch routine, a perfect way to start your day.

MORNING STRETCH ROUTINE
Length of time: 15 minutes[24]

You can start the Morning Stretch Routine while lying in bed, gradually moving to a sitting position, and eventually standing. These self-acupressure massage techniques are designed to help you begin the day with vibrancy and greater energy than you normally have. The benefits listed with each self-acupressure technique are the result of several months of daily practice.

At first, go through the Morning Stretch Routine in the order given; also try to follow the suggested times. Once you are familiar with the basic movements, feel free to improvise and change them according to your needs. For example, if you particularly enjoy massaging your legs and feet, spend extra time on them. If on the other hand, you do not enjoy or benefit from some of these exercises, feel free to delete them. You do not have to do all of these exercises. Also, you can vary the way you do each self-massage technique; for example, if you like rubbing more than pressing, feel free to make your own personal adjustments.

---

[24]*Note:* At first, this routine will take longer (approximately 30 minutes). As you get to know these exercises and their progression, you will go through them smoothly and quickly, as they flow into one another.

Head and Face

Use both of your hands to massage both sides of your face simultaneously. Lie in bed, or sit up comfortably to begin the self-acupressure routine.

1. **Head and Face Rub**
   Rub your face thoroughly from the forehead down through the eyes, nose, cheeks, jaws, lips, ears, and the back of the neck. (30 seconds)
   Rub or scratch the base of your skull to the top of your head. (10 seconds)
   Benefits: Improves the complexion, skin luster, and wrinkles.

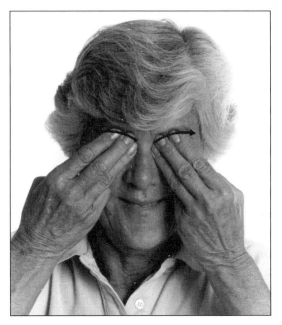

2. **Around the Eyes**
   Gently rub around the orbit of the eye. Start from the inner corner and work toward the temples. (2 times)
   Benefits: Relieves tired, sore, strained eyes.

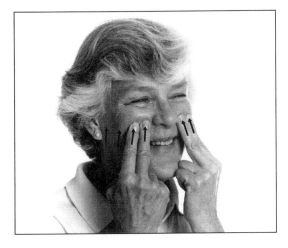

3. **Cheek Press**
   With your fingertips, press up underneath your cheekbone. Start next to
   the nose and move outward to the
   ear. (3 times) Hold the sensitive
   spots longer and take some deep
   breaths to relieve your tension or
   congestion.
   Benefits: Relieves sinus congestion,
   facial tensions, acne, earaches, and
   bleeding gums.

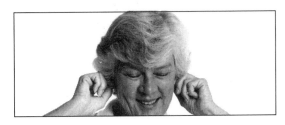

4. **Ear Massage**
   Pull your earlobes while pressing,
   rubbing and rolling the lobes. (5 seconds) Massage all the areas of your
   ear thoroughly by covering inner as
   well as outer surfaces.
   Benefits: Relieves fatigue, depression, general stress, and earaches.

5. **Skull Tap**
   Tap your fingertips over your entire
   skull. (10 seconds)
   Benefits: Stimulates growth of
   healthy hair, prevents headaches, and
   improves mental clarity.

6. **Base of Skull Press**
   Press your thumbs up underneath
   and all along the base of your skull
   with your head tilted back. This area
   may be sensitive, but continue to hold
   these spots. Take a few deep breaths.
   (10 seconds)
   Benefits: Relieves insomnia, hypertension, headaches (including migraines). Improves memory and
   alertness.

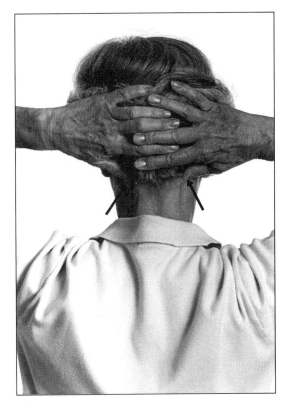

Neck

The following parts of the Daily Stretch Routine can be done while you are sitting or standing, whichever is most comfortable for you.

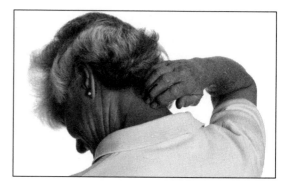

1. **Neck Rotation**
   Rotate your neck gently in each direction. (3 times)
   Benefits: Relieves anxiety, fatigue, general stress.

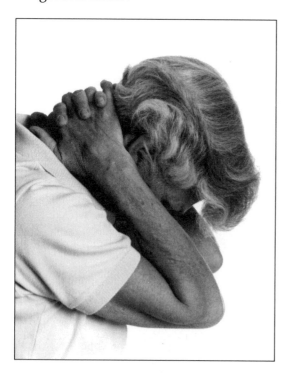

2. **Neck Squeeze**
   Interlace fingers behind your neck. Press into your neck muscles using the heels of your hands, and bring your elbows together. (3 times)
   Benefits: Relieves shoulder and neck tension, stiff neck, general stress.

3. **Neck Tap**
   Lightly tap the left side of your neck with the fingers of your right hand. Reverse sides. (5 times)
   Benefits: Relieves tiredness, lethargy, depression.

4. **Coccyx Skull Tap**
   Pat your coccyx (tailbone) with your right hand while your left hand alternately pats the base of your skull. (5 times)
   Benefits: The nervous system, especially the spine.

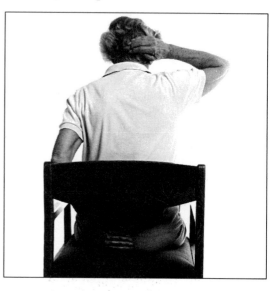

Arms and Shoulders

1. **Shoulder Rotation**
Rotate your shoulders in a circular
motion. (3 times in each direction)
Benefits: Relieves shoulder and neck
tension, uptightness, "Type A" be-
havior (aggressive, overworked, com-
pulsively goal-oriented).

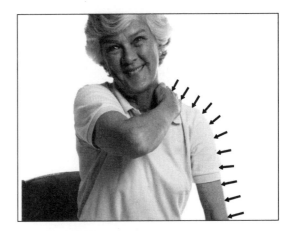

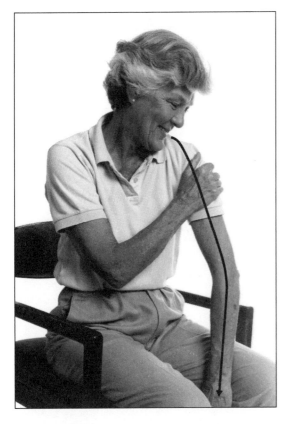

2. **Arm Rub**
Massage, knead, or rub your arms
thoroughly, going downward from
your shoulders to your hands.
(5 seconds each arm)
Benefits: Relieves poor circulation in
the hands, and fatigue.

3. **Arm and Shoulder Slap**
Gently slap from the top of your
shoulder down the arm to your hand.
(3 times each side)
Benefits: Relieves poor circulation,
chronic fatigue.

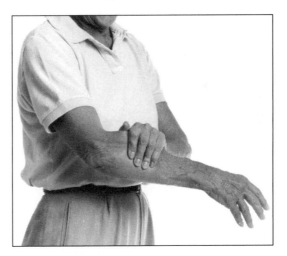

4. **Forearm Squeeze**
Knead the outer muscles of your
forearm just below your elbow.
(3 times each side)
Benefits: Upper torso, respiratory
system. Relieves depression, lethargy.

5. **Inner Elbow Massage**
   Rub your inner elbow in a circular motion with your fingertips.
   Benefits: Relieves elbow pain, hypertension, insomnia.

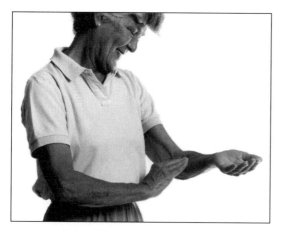

6. **Arm Swing**
   Swing your arms. (3 times)
   Benefits: Relieves poor circulation, cardiovascular conditions, insomnia.

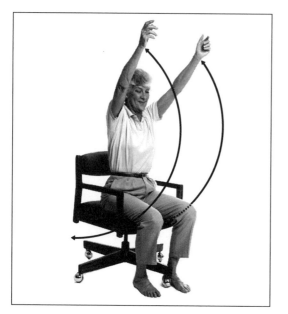

7. **Arm Stretch**
   Interlace your fingers with your hands in front of your chest. Inhale and stretch your arms directly above your head, with your palms facing up. Take a deep breath. (3 times)
   Benefits: Digestive system. Relieves shoulder tension.

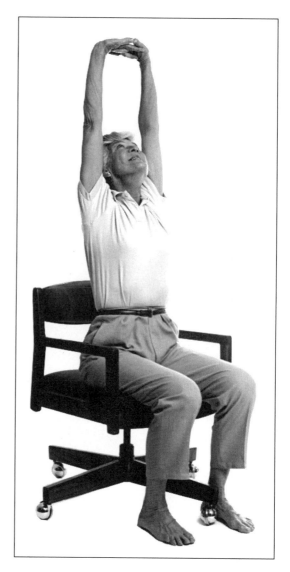

Hands and Fingers
(For preventing arthritis)

1. **Wrist Rotation**
   Rotate your wrists. (5 times)
   Benefits: Relieves wrist tendonitis, arthritis, cold hands.

2. **Finger Squeeze**
   With your left hand, squeeze each finger of your right hand from the base to the tip. Then reverse.
   (2 times each finger)
   Benefits: Relieves painful, cold hands, and hypertension.

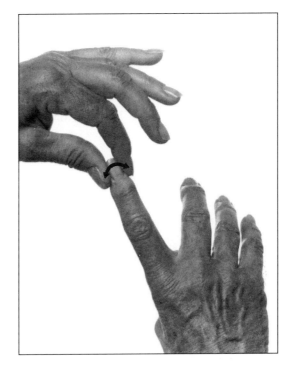

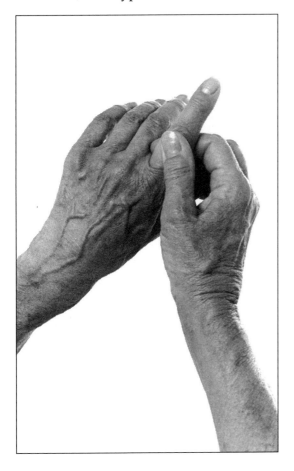

3. **Fingertip Roll**
   Squeeze and roll the fingertips of your right hand with the fingertips of your left hand. Reverse sides.
   Benefits: Relieves stiffness in the joints of the fingers.

4. **Hand Rub**
   Rub your hands together vigorously. (10 seconds) Rub the backs of your hands. (5 seconds) Use a little oil if the skin is dry.
   Benefits: Relieves poor circulation, cold hands.

5. **Hand Shake**
   Shake your hands vigorously. (5 seconds)
   Benefits: Improves circulation into the hands.

6. **Hand Clap**
   Clap your hands. (5 times)
   Benefits: Circulatory and nervous systems.

7. **Finger Bend**
   Gently bend back each finger and the thumb of your right hand with your left hand. Reverse.
   Benefits: Improves circulation in the hands.

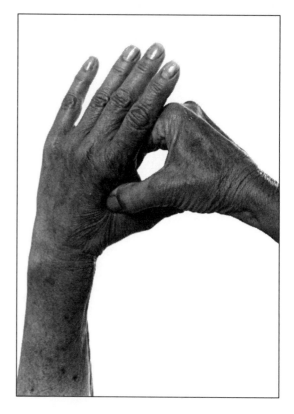

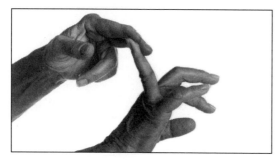

8. **Hand Massage**
   Massage the palm of your hand thoroughly with your opposite hand, pressing with your thumb. Massage into the webbing between each finger. (15 seconds on each hand)
   Benefits: The hand reflexology points corresponding to all parts of the body. See the chart on page 75.

9. **Web Press**
   Firmly press the webbing of each hand between your thumb and index finger. (5 seconds on each side)
   Benefits: Relieves headaches, toothaches, arthritic pains, and sinus problems.

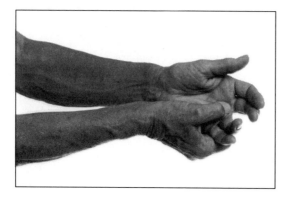

Pelvis and Spine
(While standing)

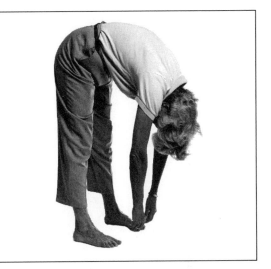

1. **Pelvic Rotation**
   Rotate your pelvis in each direction with your hands on your hips. Start very slowly if lower back problems exist. (3 times)
   Benefits: Relieves frustration, helps prevent sciatica. Improves waistline; increases energy and circulation through the legs.

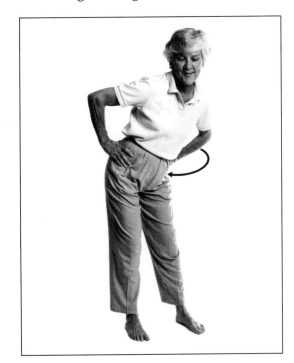

2. **Rag Doll**
   Bend forward and hang like a rag doll; then bend backward arching your back and using your hands to support your lower back. (3 times)
   Benefits: Kidneys, urinary system. Relieves lower back problems.

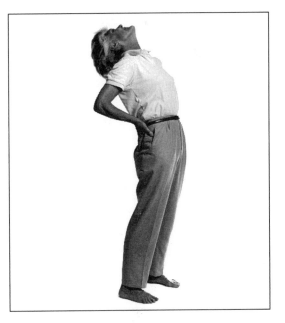

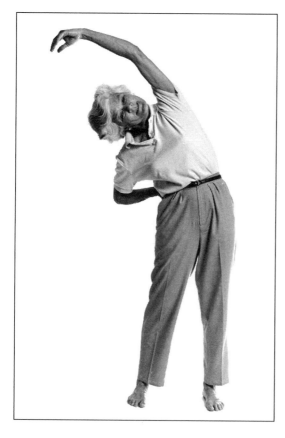

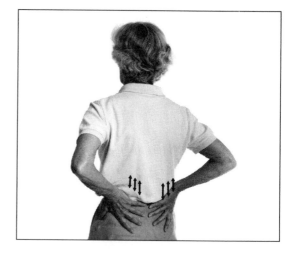

5. **Sacrum Rub**
Rub up and down at the base of your spine on either side using your thumb knuckles. (10 seconds)
Benefits: Urinary system. Relieves lower back pain, hemorrhoids, sciatica.

3. **Bamboo in the Wind**
Raise your left arm and sway to the right, keeping your back straight. Reverse sides. (4 times)
Benefits: Improves posture, flexibility of the spine.

4. **Lower Back Massage**
Rub the lower back area using the palms of both hands. (10 seconds) Rock and press both fists into your lower back, 2 or 3 inches from your spine. (10 seconds)
Benefits: Kidneys, and general stamina. Relieves ringing in the ears, lower backaches.

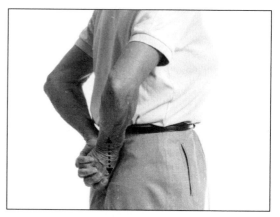

6. **Buttocks Pound**
Make a fist with both of your hands, and pound your buttocks thoroughly. (10 seconds)
Benefits: Relieves pelvic tension, constipation, frustration.

Torso
(Sitting in a comfortable, straight-back chair)

1. **Chest Drum***
   Tap the upper chest muscles (located just below the collarbone) thoroughly, using both fists. (10 seconds)
   Benefits: Relieves chest congestion, respiratory problems, anxiety.
   Caution: Avoid this exercise if you have heart or lung disease.

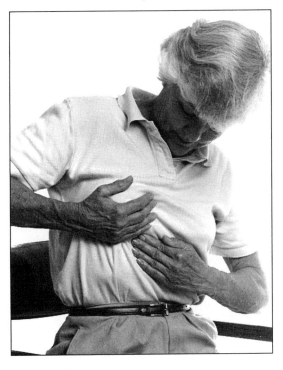

2. **Breast Massage**
   Gently move the breast tissue to the side or center and massage the muscle under the breast.
   (5 seconds on each side)
   Benefits: Relieves heartburn, chest pain, palpitations.

3. **Rib Massage**
   Using your left hand, massage in between the ribs on your right side. Start from the breastbone and move outward. Then reverse. (10 seconds)
   Benefits: Digestive system. Relieves side aches, gas, and belching; increases the vital capacity of the lungs.

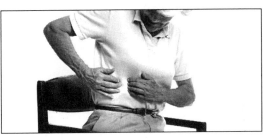

4. **Sternum Tap***
   Using the fingertips of both hands, tap down the center of your chest along your breastbone (sternum) (3 times)
   Benefits: Cardiovascular system. Relieves heartburn, anxiety, nervousness, difficulty breathing, chest tightness.

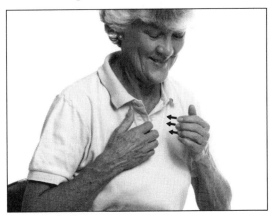

Caution: People with pacemakers should not do this exercise.

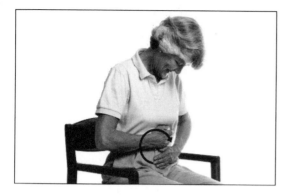

5. **Tummy Rub**
Rub your stomach and abdomen area clockwise (as you are looking at the abdomen) using both hands. (10 seconds)
Benefits: Abdominal organs. Relieves constipation, abdominal distension.

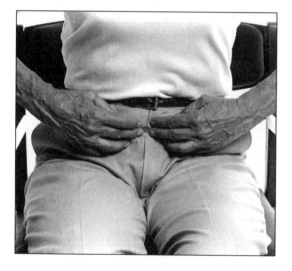

6. **Below the Navel Press**
Press two inches below your navel with the fingertips of both hands. (5 seconds)
Benefits: Elimination, urinary system, vitality.

Legs
(Sitting in a comfortable, straight-back chair)

1. **Leg Rub**
Rub or knead your legs from your upper thighs to your feet using both hands. (30 seconds)
Benefits: Relieves leg pain or numbness, stiffness, leg cramps.

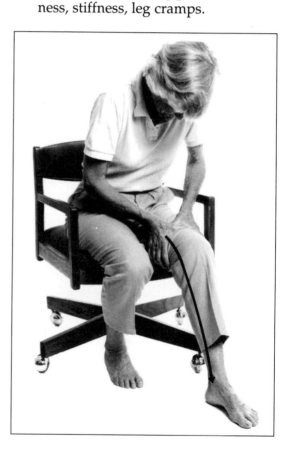

2. **Calf Press**

Place both thumbs in back of one knee. Press in slowly for 3 seconds and release. Then move down the calf to the ankle, pressing every inch as you descend. (once each side)
Benefits: Relieves spasms in calf muscle, lower backaches, knee pain.

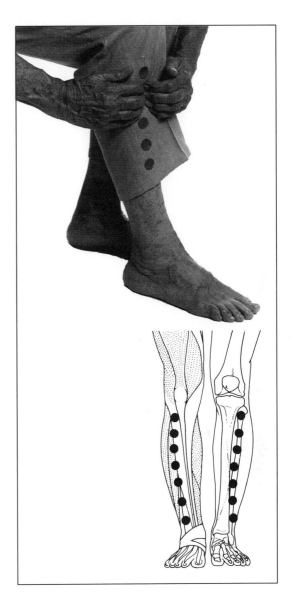

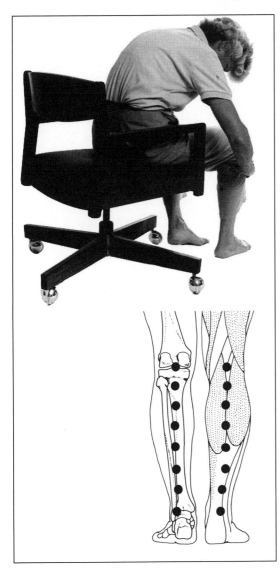

3. **Shin Press**

Using the fingertips of both hands, press on the outside of the shin bone, moving down toward the foot. (once each side)
Benefits: Relieves physical exhaustion, digestive disorders, shin splints.

Feet and Ankles

(While sitting with socks removed, work on one foot at a time.)

1. **Toe Massage**
   Roll each toe. (2 seconds each)
   Bend each toe back and forth.
   (2 seconds each)
   Benefits: Eyes, ears, nose, and throat.
   Improves circulation; relieves sinus problems.

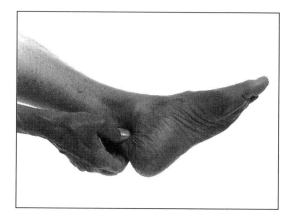

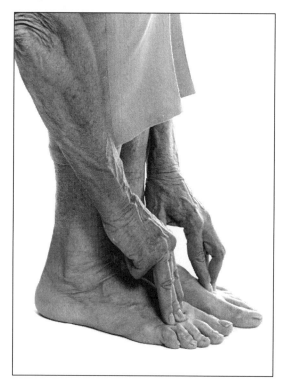

3. **Ankle Press**
   Inner ankle: Press the inner ankle with your thumbs, working in a circular motion. (10 seconds)
   Outer ankle: Rub your outer ankle with your fingertips. (5 seconds)
   Benefits: Urinary system. Relieves ankle pain.

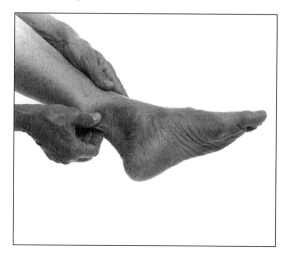

2. **Top of Foot Massage**
   Using your fingertips, press into the webbing between each toe and massage in between the bones on the tops of your feet. (10 seconds)
   Benefits: Digestive system. Relieves allergies and tired, aching feet.

4. **Achilles Tendon**
   Squeeze and knead the Achilles tendon area. (3 times)
   Benefits: Relieves edema, swollen ankles, foot pain, rheumatism.

5. **Arch Massage**
    Press the arch of the foot with your
    thumbs, beginning at the heel and
    moving toward the large toe. (2 times)
    Benefits: Spine, digestive system,
    hypoglycemia.

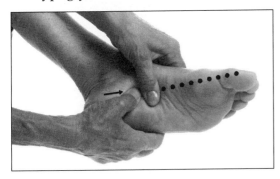

6. **Bottom of Foot Press**
    Press all the areas of the bottom of the
    foot with your thumbs. Finish by
    massaging the entire foot.
    (30 seconds)
    Benefits: All of the internal organs.

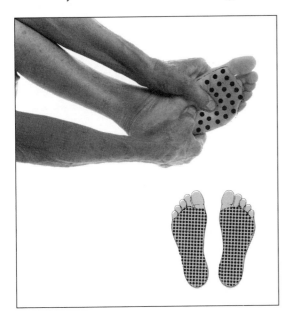

MIDDAY REFRESHER

Length of time: 5 minutes

This series of self-acupressure exercises is designed to provide midday revitalization and relaxation. Many people spend long hours sitting at desks or in cars, accumulating tension; in addition, muscles that aren't being used properly tend to atrophy. Instead of allowing built-up tension and under-used muscles to aggravate your arthritis, use this midday refresher to help you break your daily patterns. You can do this routine at the office or at home — while sitting in a chair — in only five minutes. You can also incorporate this set into a midday exercise program for optimal performance and enjoyment. And you can do the routine any time to feel better, less pressured, and more alert.

For the following exercises, sit comfortably in a chair.

1. **Shoulder Hook**
   Use your right hand to squeeze your left shoulder. (15 seconds) Switch sides and squeeze. (15 seconds)
   Benefits: Relieves shoulder tension and pain, impatience, fatigue.

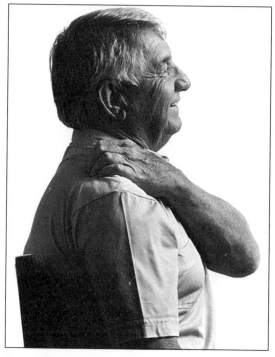

2. **Elbow Lift**
   Place your hands on your shoulders: Right hand on right shoulder, left hand on left shoulder, elbows out to the sides. Inhale and lift your elbows up and toward each other. Exhale as you relax down. (3 times)
   Benefits: Relieves depression, aching shoulders, stiff neck, general stress.

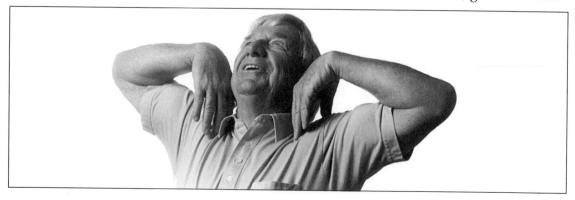

3. **Neck Press**
Interlace your fingers behind your neck. Bring your elbows in toward each other. Take three deep breaths through your nose while remaining in this position.
Benefits: Relieves stiff neck, headaches, hypertension.

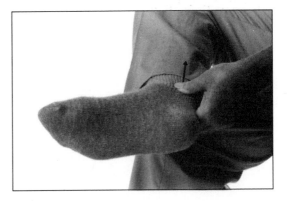

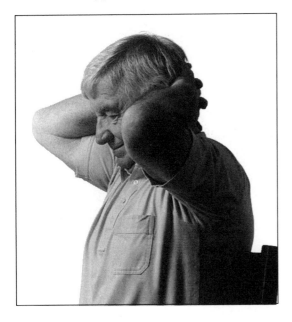

6. **Ankle Press**
Squeeze the Achilles tendon from the base of the calf to the ankle. (twice on each side)
Benefits: Relieves lower back pain, ankle pain, ringing in the ears.

7. **Leg Press**
Cross your legs and firmly squeeze from below your knee to your ankle. (3 times on each leg)
Benefits: Relieves leg cramps, stiffness, edema, varicose veins.

4. **Neck Rotations**
Slowly rotate your head in a clockwise direction as you breathe deeply. Then rotate counterclockwise. (2 or 3 times slowly in each direction)
Benefits: Relieves nervousness, anxiety, general stress, hypertension.

5. **Joint Rotations**
Rotate your hands on your wrists while you rotate your feet on your ankles. (10 seconds)
Benefits: Relieves joint pain and stiffness.

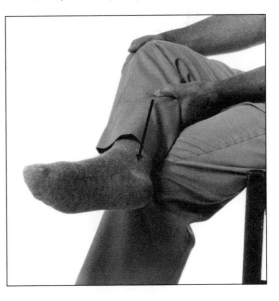

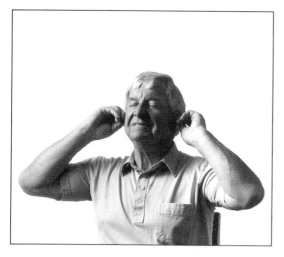

8. **Ear Press**
Massage and press all parts of your ears, preferably while keeping your eyes closed. (30 seconds)
Benefits: Well-being for the entire body.

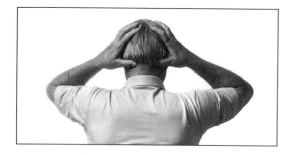

9. **Base of Skull Press**
Use your thumbs to press underneath the base of the skull. Tilt your head back and press upward. Take three long, deep breaths as you press. (15 seconds)
Benefits: Relieves insomnia, hypertension, headaches (including migraines). Improves memory and alertness.

10. **Shoulder and Hand Shake**
Shake your shoulders. (10 seconds) Then vigorously shake your hands. (5 seconds)
Benefits: Improves circulatory system; relieves shoulder tension.

11. **Hand Rub**
Rub your hands together to create heat. (5 to 10 seconds)
Benefits: Relieves cold hands.

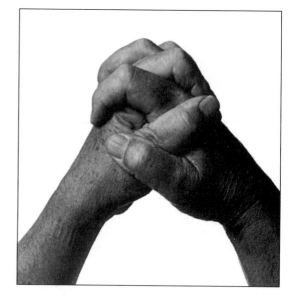

12. **Hand Squeeze**
Interlace your fingers and squeeze. (3 times)
Benefits: Increased circulation and well-being.

EVENING RELAXATION
Suggested Duration: 10 minutes

After a full day of activities, we often feel drained and sometimes even irritable. Frequently, we bring home with us many of the day's pressures and problems. The evening routine is designed to help you feel more at ease. This series is somewhat different from the morning and midday routines in that it involves quiet, gentle touching and holding of points for longer periods of time. Many people find that simply touching the following acupressure points for long periods of time helps them to deeply relax.

The evening routine can be done before dinner or at least an hour after dinner, once you've had time to digest your food. Many people prefer to do this routine in bed just before going to sleep. The ensuing relaxation relieves arthritic discomforts, helps them to sleep more deeply, and results in their feeling more alert when they wake up in the morning.

Practice this routine as presented here. After you become more familiar with each of the following acupressure points (illustrated in the next few pages), adapt it to your own personal style and preferences. For example, many people enjoy doing the Head Heart Touch (see p. 64) in bed for several minutes before going to sleep. A calm, relaxed state of mind is conducive to pain relief and helps reinforce a positive outlook on life. Do the following routine while lying down or sitting in a comfortable chair. Begin with three long, deep breaths.

1. **Shoulder Touch**
Lightly squeeze your shoulders. (30 seconds)
Benefits: Relieves shoulder tension, uptightness, irritability.

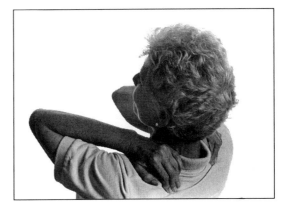

2. **Neck Touch**
Interlace your fingers behind your neck. Use the heels of your hands to press into your neck muscles, bringing your elbows together. (3 times) Continue to hold lightly. (30 seconds)
Benefits: Relieves stiff neck, headaches, hypertension.

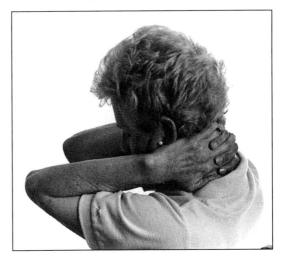

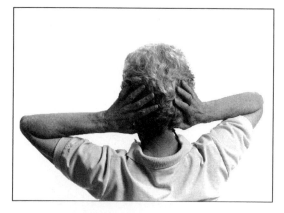

Place your fingers on your temples. Lightly rub in a circular motion. (15 seconds) Hold lightly for another 15 seconds.
Benefits: Relieves eyestrain, headaches; improves memory, concentration.

3. **Base of Skull Touch**
Use your thumbs to press underneath the base of your skull. Tilt your head back and press upward. If these points feel painful or sore, hold lightly. (30 seconds)
Benefits: Relieves insomnia, hypertension, headaches (including migraines). Improves memory and alertness.

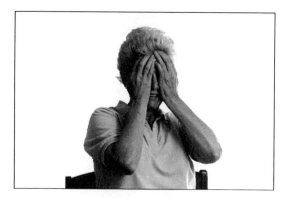

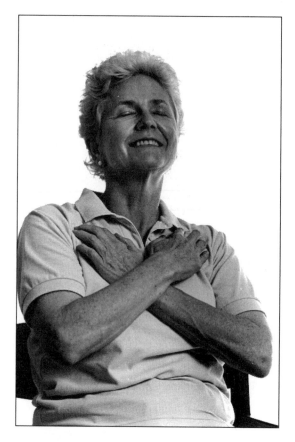

4. **Eye Temple Touch**
Close your eyes. Place your palms over your eyes with your fingers lightly touching your forehead. Allow your eyes to relax. (1 minute) If your eyes are tired or sore, extend this for 3 to 5 minutes.

5. **Upper Chest Touch**
Cross your arms, place your fingertips below your collar bone, and hold. Close your eyes and feel yourself breathing. (1 minute)
Benefits: High blood pressure. Relieves anxiety, asthma, chest congestion.

6. **Solar Plexus Touch**
Interlace your fingers as shown, and place them over your solar plexus. (1 minute)
Benefits: Relieves indigestion, heartburn, ulcers.

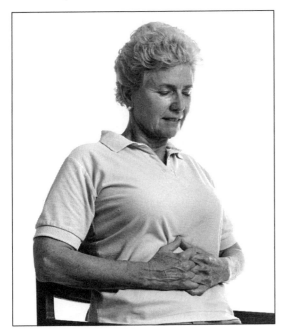

7. **Spine Touch**
Place your right hand at the base of your spine. Place your left hand between the big vertebrae where the neck joins the shoulders. (30 seconds) Keep your right hand at the base of the spine. Move your left hand to the base of your skull. (hold 30 seconds)
Benefits: Central nervous system, spinal column, vitality.

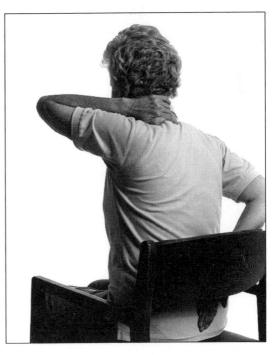

8. **Head Heart Touch**
   Place your right hand on the top of
   your head. Place your left hand over
   the center of your chest.
   (hold 1 minute)
   Benefits: Relieves nervousness, anxiety, impatience, aggravation.

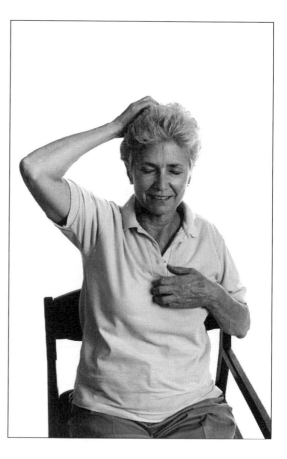

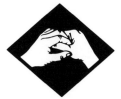

CHAPTER VI

PAIN
RELIEF FOR
SPECIFIC AREAS

PAIN
RELIEF FOR
SPECIFIC AREAS

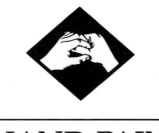

HAND PAIN

The most common area for arthritis is the hands. Few joints in the body are as important to our daily activities as the joints in the hand, and when our fingers are disabled, we are profoundly and adversely affected. In rheumatoid arthritis, the inflamed knuckles usually deteriorate, accompanied by muscular wasting, resulting in joint and finger deformities. However, after many months of regularly practicing the daily routines and acupressure massage exercises that follow, you can improve the condition of your arthritic joints.

Acupressure, along with hand exercise and rest, can help prevent arthritic destruction of the knuckles, keep the joints stabilized, and minimize abnormal pressures in the knuckles. These hand exercises and self-acupressure methods can also strengthen the tendons and muscles to allow greater use of your fingers, with less pain and discomfort. Combining hand motions, such as flexions and rotations, with acupressure point stimulation will result in increased effectiveness.

A recent client of mine, with a history of arthritis, injured herself while trying to open a jar of pickles. Her wrist became so inflamed and painful that her use of that entire hand was inhibited. Her pain radiated out from the wrist into her fingers and spread into her forearm and up into her elbow joint.

When I examined her arm during our first session, her joints were inflamed and so stiff that I had my doubts whether acupressure could be effective. As I held her acupressure points and gently mani-

pulated the joints in her hand and wrist, the stiffness gradually eased. But this increase in flexibility did not last long at first. It took about six weekly visits for the acupressure sessions to have lasting effects. I attribute a great deal of our success with acupressure to her efforts to heal herself by regularly practicing the arthritis relief hand techniques that are contained in this chapter.

Another client of mine came to me after she had attempted to refinish her coffee table. On a cold, rainy day on her back porch, she finally finished the job by spray painting the table. Unfortunately, her index finger had become inflamed and painful from holding the button of the spray can. I met her several months later at a community senior citizens center where I was teaching a group of senior citizens how to use self-acupressure to relieve arthritic pain. Her hand was slightly discolored, her fingers stiffly bent, and her joints inflamed and gnarled.

The next week, she complained that these techniques seemed to aggravate her pain. In response, I explained to the group that these "flare-ups," although discouraging, are common and often an important part of working out the constrictions that are at the root of joint degeneration and inflammation. I encouraged her to hold points directly on the painful joints for several minutes at a time, particularly Point #1 in the webbing between the thumb and index finger, after running warm water over her hands for a few minutes.

Several weeks later, she came to me

with a glowing report that ninety percent of her pain was gone. She now felt equipped to deal with any further flare-ups.

With persistent, daily practice of these simple self-help techniques, you can relieve your arthritic pain, increase your circulation, and prevent other joints from developing arthritis. In order to protect the vulnerable joints of your hands, you will learn how to use your hand in positions that place minimal stress on the joints. If you want to keep fingers flexible and strong as well as relieve your pain, you must practice the points and one set of hand exercises or self-massage techniques at least once or twice a day.

Each of the following points should be held for one minute each with firm, steady pressure. Use whatever finger, thumb, or knuckle makes it easy to gradually apply firm, deep pressure into each of these points. Hold the points that feel directly related to your arthritic joint pains for two or three minutes longer to help relieve the pain.

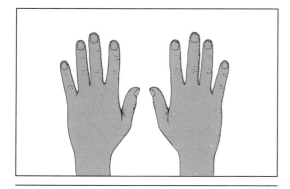

[25] These numbers refer to the acupuncture/acupressure point system of the body. You do not need to know any of these reference numbers to practice the Arthritis Relief Program.

HAND PAIN RELIEF POINTS[25]

TW 4 is located in the center of the outside of the wrist joint in an indentation.
Benefits: Relieves wrist pain, carpal tunnel syndrome, wrist joint arthritis, inability to grasp objects, wrist weakness, forearm and elbow pain, swollen wrist, inability to flex or extend.

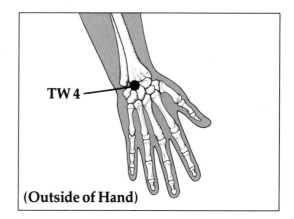

(Outside of Hand)

LI 5 is located in the hollow of the wrist joint near the webbing between the thumb and index finger.
Benefits: Relieves arthritic pains in the bones or joints that attach to the thumb or index finger, wrist joint pain.

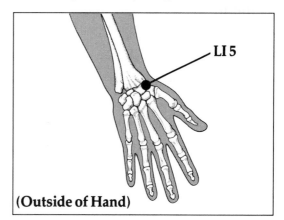

(Outside of Hand)

H 7 is located on the inside of the wrist crease below the inside center of the little finger.
Benefits: Relieves wrist pain and insomnia. This point is also traditionally used for cardiac disorders.

P 7 is located in the middle of the inside wrist crease.
Benefits: Relieves arthritic pain in the palm or middle finger, appetite imbalance, emotional imbalances, trauma, and insomnia.

L 9 is located in the hollow on the inside wrist crease directly below the base of the thumb.
Benefits: Relieves wrist and arm pain, anxiety, and insomnia.

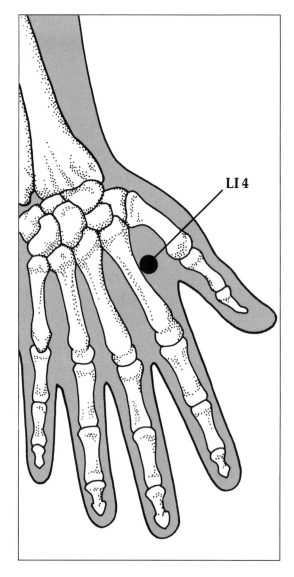

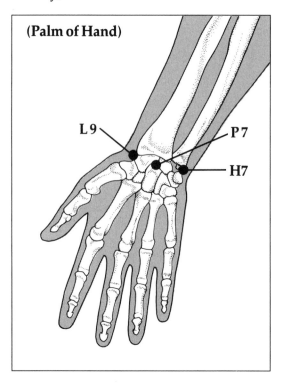

(Palm of Hand)

L 9   P 7   H7

Point #1 is located in the webbing between the index and thumb, close to the metacarpal bone that attaches to the index finger.
Benefits: This an important pain point for the hands, arms, and head. It is also an anti-inflammatory point helpful for relieving most headaches.

RANGE OF MOTION EXERCISES

The hand stretching exercises contained in this section are useful for assessing the flexibility your fingers, hands and wrists, and are also remedial methods of increasing the range of motion of the joints. If you find that your hand movements are especially difficult or painful, then it is necessary to work at increasing the flexibility of the joint through acupressure and daily hand stretching exercises.

As you practice the following hand exercises, make a note in your arthritis journal (see pages 205-216) of any pain you develop, what type of pain it is, and exactly where it occurs. Use the following suggestions if you do have pain while practicing any of these range of motion stretching exercises.

Suggestions

1. Stop just before the point of pain.
2. Locate the painful site by applying firm pressure on it with your other hand.
3. Contract the muscles in your hand or wrist for a few seconds as you hold the painful point. Relax and repeat the contraction several times.
4. Gently move your hand in order to relax it, and take slow, deep breaths for a few minutes.
5. Again, try the same range of motion exercise, but very slowly. If you feel some relief but the pain is still present, then repeat the above procedure again. If the range of motion makes your pain even worse, then discon-

tinue the exercise, rest the joint, and see a physical therapist or doctor for further advice.

EASY HAND EXERCISES

Wrist Flexes

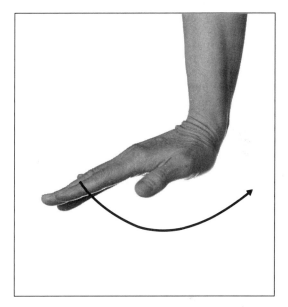

1. Extend your hand upward to stretch your wrist and fingers.
2. Flex your hand downward, bringing the palm of your hand closer to the inside of your wrist.
3. Continue to flex your wrists in both directions to increase flexibility.

Turning Hands Over

1. Place both of your palms face down on the top of a desk or table.
2. Turn your hands over, placing the backs of your hands on the table.
3. Take slow, deep breaths as you continue to turn your hands over several times.

Nodding Hand

1. Tuck the thumb into the palm of your hand and cover it with your fingers by making a fist.
2. Turn your fist so that the back of your first thumb knuckle is facing up.
3. Extend your arm straight out in front of you without bending your elbow.

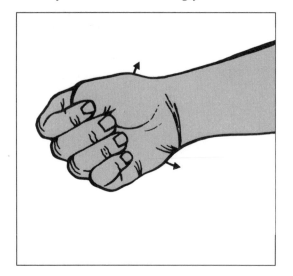

4. Keeping your arm stationary, very slowly move your hand up and down. When you flex your fist down, you should feel a stretch in the base of your thumb.
5. Repeat this nodding hand motion several times. Gradually increase the number of times you do this exercise.

Note: If you have pain when you move your hand downward in this exercise, then you are flexing your hand down too fast. Move your hand much slower and hold it down a few seconds longer. This stretch can be very helpful for relieving arthritis hand pain.

Hand Windshield Wipers

1. Place your hands on the top of a table with your palms facing down

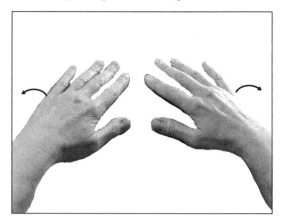

2. Turn both of your hands inward, bringing your fingertips closer together.
3. Turn both of your hands outward.
4. Continue to slowly turn your hands inward and outward.

Hand Spread

1. Extend your fingers straight.
2. Spread your fingers apart for several seconds to gently stretch your hand.
3. Relax your hands down into your lap and take a deep breath.

Hand Rotations

1. Gently shake your hands to promote circulation and to relax them.
2. Slowly rotate both of your hands on your wrists four or five times.
3. Circle your hands four or five times in the opposite direction as you take a couple of slow, long, deep breaths.

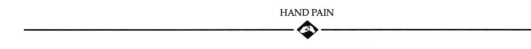

HAND REFLEXOLOGY CHART

Arthritis and other health imbalances in a particular area of the body often register in corresponding areas of the hand. This chart illustrates these areas. Pressure on these reflexology points or zones can accomplish two goals: relieving your hand pain locally, and also stimulating the associated nerves to help relieve arthritic pain and inflammation in related areas of the body.

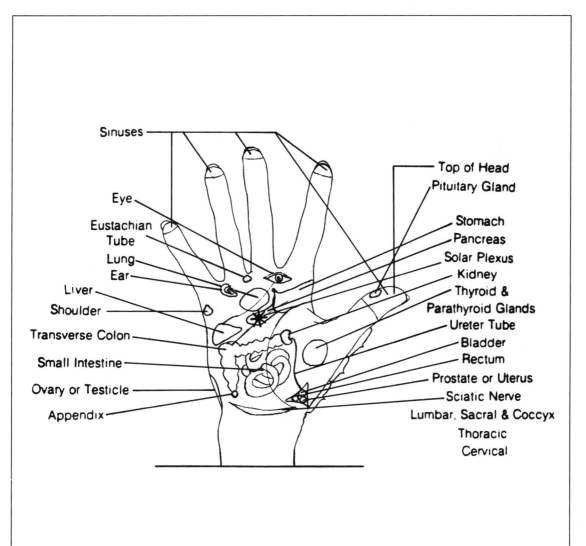

ACUPRESSURE POINT CHART

The following chart illustrates all of the acupressure points on the hand. Use this chart to find the points that seem directly related or closest to your pain, as well as other corresponding points that are nearby the painful site. Explore these points as you practice the hand massage. This acupressure chart will help you to find these key trigger points that help to relieve arthritis.

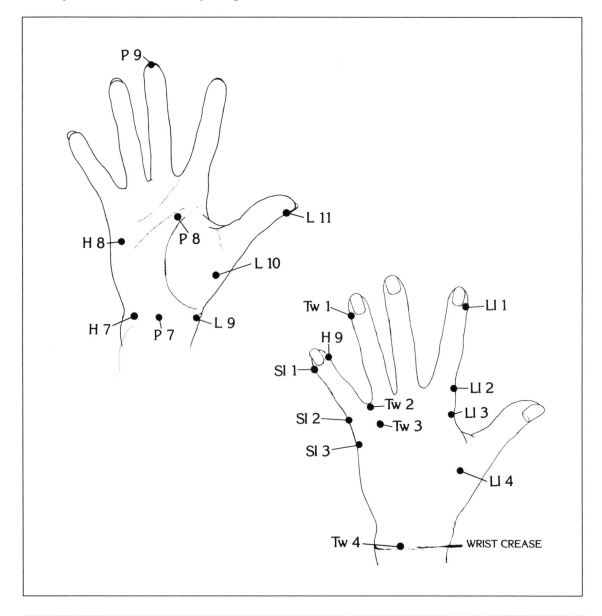

EIGHT DAILY SELF-MASSAGE EXERCISES

1. **Wrist Rotation**
   Slowly rotate your hands around on your wrists. Circulate five times in one direction, then five times in the other direction.
   Suggestion: It helps to take deep breaths as you do the wrist rotation.
   Variation: Rotate your hands on your wrists more rapidly to stimulate an increase in circulation.

2. **Finger Squeeze**
   With your left hand, squeeze each

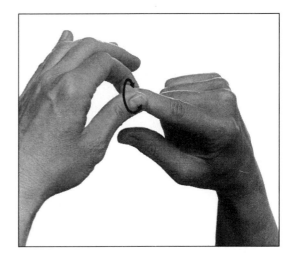

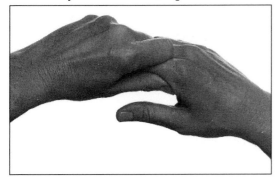

finger of your right hand three times, moving from the base to the top of the finger. Repeat each finger again. Then change hands and use the same procedure on the fingers of the left hand. Again, repeat each finger.
Suggestion: Elongate or stretch each finger by firmly pulling your fingers outward.
Variation: Vibrate each finger by rapidly rolling your fingers at the joint where you would squeeze. (The next fingertip self-massage describes this technique in greater depth.)

3. **Fingertip Roll**
   Squeeze and gently twist each finger of your right hand back and forth with the fingertips of your left hand. Grasp the points (illustrated) at the

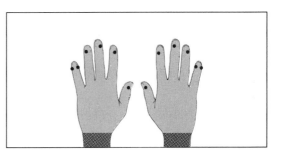

base of the nail, using the thumbs and index finger of your working hand. Then briskly roll the fingertip, creating a vibrating effect to stimulate circulation.
   Now repeat the fingertip roll on your other hand. Grasp the fingertips of your left hand with your right hand. Again, briskly roll each fingertip, creating a vibrating effect to increase your circulation.

4. **Hand Rub**
   Vigorously rub the palms of your hands together for about ten seconds to create heat. Rub the back of one hand with the palm of your other hand. Then reverse, rubbing the back of your other hand.
   Suggestion: Use firm pressure between your hands to create friction as you rub them together.
   Variation: Rub your hands together for 10 to 20 seconds, one over the other as if you were washing your hands with soap.

5. **Hand and Shoulder Shake** (10 to 30 seconds) Shake out both of your hands, letting them move freely on your wrists. Slowly begin to exaggerate the hand shake by letting your arms and shoulders gently shake with your hands to free the circulation.
   Suggestion: When you do this exercise, let your arms hang down by your sides with your shoulders relaxed downward.
   Variation: After shaking, "give yourself a hand" by clapping your hands together several times.

6. **Finger Rotations**
   Use your opposite hand to gently stretch each of your fingers in a slow rotating motion. Emphasize the rotation of your thumbs, along with deep breathing through your nose, to overcome sluggishness, depression, and fatigue.
   Suggestion: Repeat the finger rotations at least two or three times a day to maximize your joint flexibility.

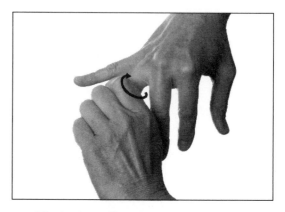

Variation: First massage the base of the finger and then rotate the finger to further increase the range of motion.

7. **Finger Traction** (5 seconds per finger) Pull each of your fingers outward, gently twisting each finger away from you as you pull. Twist the thumbs toward you to pull in harmony with the structure of the hands.

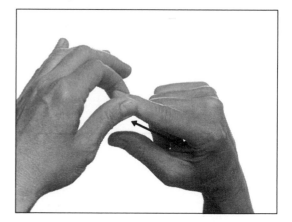

Suggestion: Firmly stretch each finger by giving five to ten seconds of steady traction.
Variation: Squeeze each joint of the finger, starting with the base and sliding outward to the top of the finger.

8. **Finger Bend** (10 seconds per finger)
Gently bend back each finger of your right hand, one finger at a time. Next,

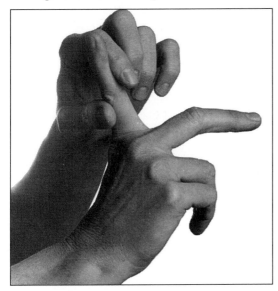

stretch each of your fingers down toward the palm of your hand. Press down on the three bones of the finger, stretching each of the joints. Reverse to work on your left hand.

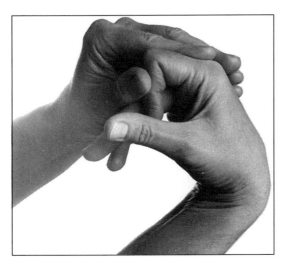

Suggestion: Gradually apply pressure to stretch the fingers backward. Slowly increase the amount of time you hold the stretch.

Variation: Interlace your fingers with your palms facing each other. Turn the palms outward and stretch fingers by straightening your arms out in front of you. Release the stretch and gently shake out your hands. Repeat the stretch and the shake-out a few more times.

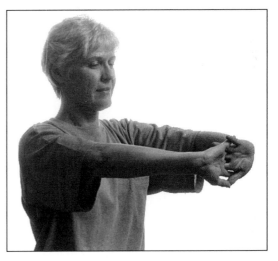

THE COMPLETE SELF-MASSAGE HAND ROUTINE

Warming the Hands

Position: Place the palms of your hands together.
Directions:
1. Apply a moderate amount of pressure between your palms.
2. Rub your hands together briskly for a minute to create a heat.
3. Interlace your fingers with the palms facing each other. Squeeze your fingertips against the back of your hands. Firmly hold for five seconds.

Relax your hands as you take a long, deep breath. Repeat the hand squeeze rhythmically for a minute.
Suggestions: Try putting a few drops of vegetable oil (like almond or coconut oil) on your hands before rubbing them. This will further help increase the generation of heat when the friction is created. Immediately after rubbing your hands together to create a heat, place the palms of your hands over your closed eyes. Feel the energy absorbing for a minute. Then slowly massage your entire face, covering the temples, bridge of the nose, and underneath the base of the skull. Lastly, massage your ears with your eyes closed.

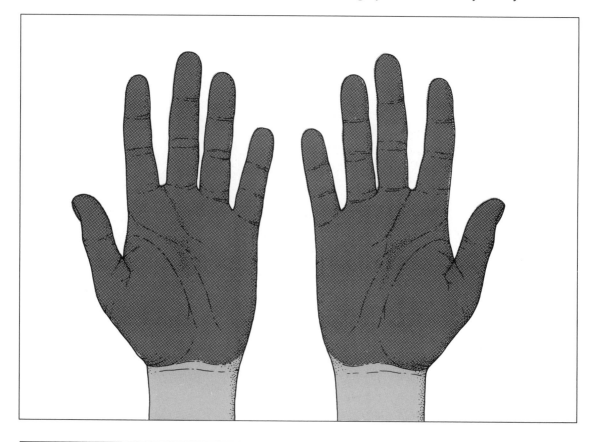

Finger Press I

Position: Open the hand you want to work on with your fingers comfortably stretched out. Place the fingers of your working hand in back of your receiving hand, and keep your working thumb in front.

Directions:
1. Press into each of the points illustrated.
2. Progress in rows, starting at the tip of each finger.
3. Hold each point for about five seconds. Release and slide your fingers to the next point.

Suggestion: Spend extra time working around your tight or painful joints. You may repeat this finger press three or four times a day.

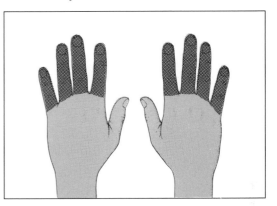

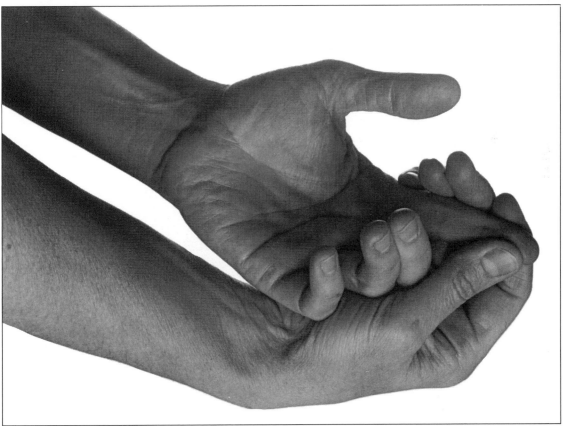

Finger Press II

Position: Turn your hand so that your palm is facing down. Grasp the sides of each finger with your working hand.

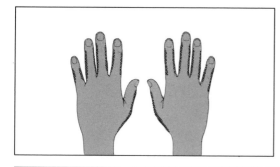

Directions:
1. Thoroughly press into the sides of each finger, holding each position for about five seconds.
2. Start at the base of the finger and move slowly toward the nail.
3. Focus on working in the joints where the finger bends, as well as on pressing the base of the nail.

Suggestion: Try gently pulling each finger outward as you progress from the base to the fingertip. Roll each finger as you apply pressure to increase the circulation.

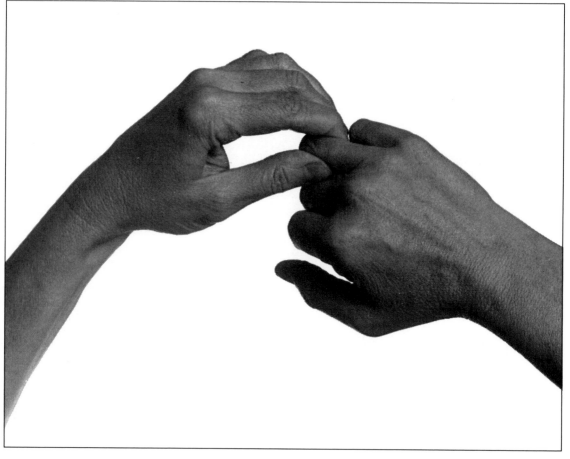

Finger Joint Press

Position: Place your thumb on one side and your fingers on the other side of whatever finger you want to work on.
Directions:
1. Carefully but firmly press into the joints of each finger.
2. Press around the base of each nail.
3. Go back to the worst joints. Hold directly on the painful points with lighter pressure but without releasing until you feel the pain subside.
4. Gradually release the pressure and go on to another painful joint.

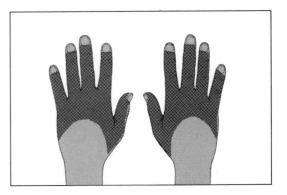

Suggestion: Roll each finger (one at a time) back and forth to increase your circulation. Alternate between working on your right and left hands to help make this less tiring.

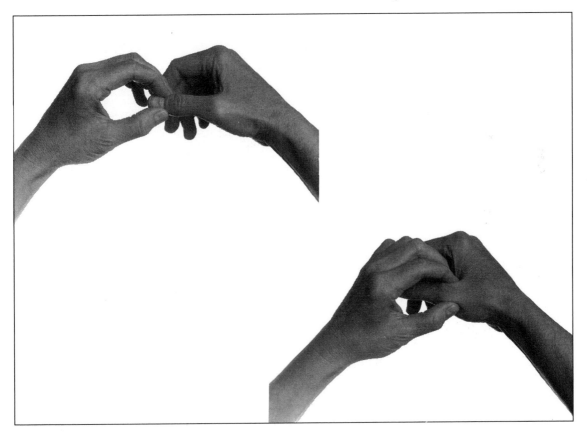

Finger Webbing

Position: Place your working thumb on the palm of your other hand with your fingers wrapped around the outside of the hand. Position your thumb and fingers opposite each other to work in the webbing between the base of the finger.

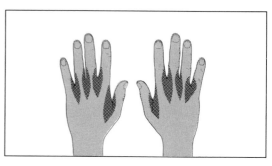

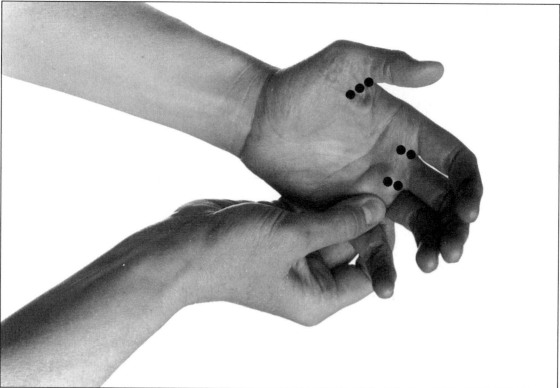

Directions:

1. Clamp into the webbing for 30 to 60 seconds for each finger.
2. Rub with firm pressure, working in between the bones.
3. If time permits, repeat the finger webbing. This time rub much slower and press slightly deeper.

Suggestion: If you find a point that is particularly sore, hold directly on the spot with less pressure until the pain subsides. Although it may hurt while you massage the webbed areas of the hand, this stimulation often brings great relief from arthritic pain and stiffness.

Outer Hand Massage

Position: Place your fingers in between the bones on the top of the hand. Position your thumb on the palm of the hand to be worked on.

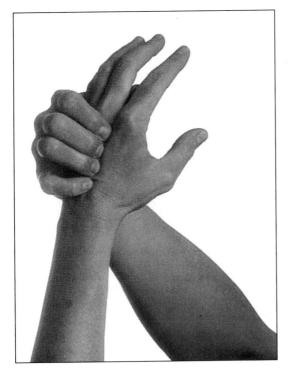

Directions:
1. Press into the indentations between the bones on the top of the hand.
2. Slide the fingers along the troughs starting between the knuckles. Using firm pressure, slide your fingertips along the grooves toward your wrists.
3. Return to the areas that are most sore. Hold directly on the most painful points in the troughs with steady prolonged pressure (without moving). Continue to hold until you feel the pain subside.

Suggestion: With your fingers in the troughs on the outside of the hand, slowly rotate your hand on the wrist. Remember to breathe deeply. Also, stimulate the anti-inflammatory Point #1

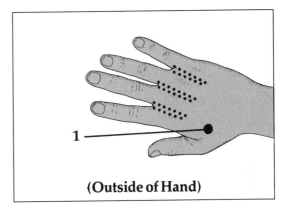

(Outside of Hand)

by placing your working thumb between your other thumb and index finger. Place the fingertips of your working hand on the outside portion of the hand being worked on. Use your thumb to stimulate Point #1, working underneath the bone that attaches to your index finger.

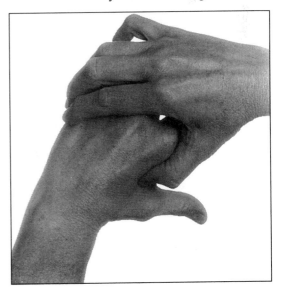

Side Squeeze

Position: Place the palm of your working hand over the top of your receiving hand. Curve the fingers of your working hand with the fingertips touching the palm of the hand being worked on.

Directions:

1. Gradually press into the top of the hand for five seconds at a time using the heel of your working hand. Knead different parts of your hand for about a minute.
2. Use your fingertips to grasp the fleshy portion of the side of your hand at the base of your little finger.
3. Firmly press the center of the inside of your wrist with your fingertips as the heel of your hand presses the center of the outside of your wrist.

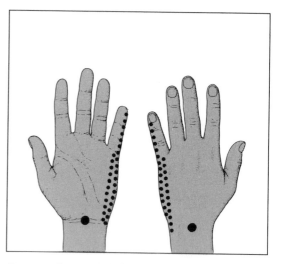

Suggestion: Hold the inner and outer points in the center of the wrist crease for a minute or two. These points are excellent for relieving arthritis in the wrists and fingers.

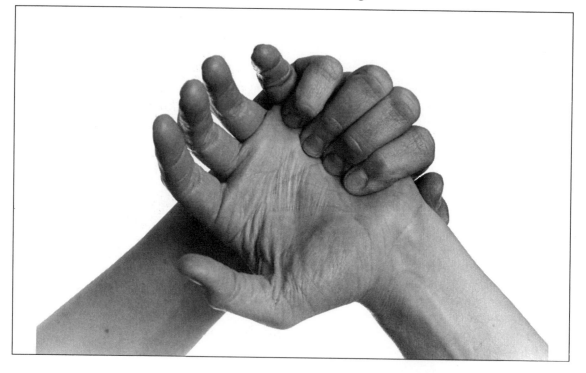

Thumb Press

Position: Place the thumb to be worked on in the palm of the working hand.

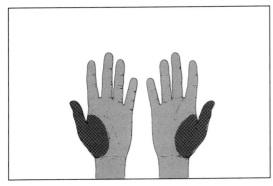

Directions:

1. Use all your fingers to press into your thumb for three to five seconds.

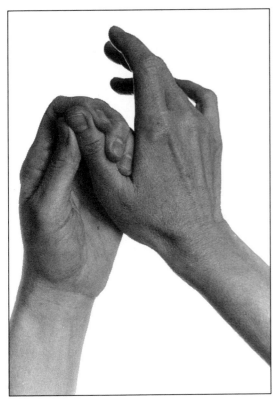

2. Squeeze and knead the base of the thumb in a pumping fashion.
3. Firmly massage into the thumb joints.

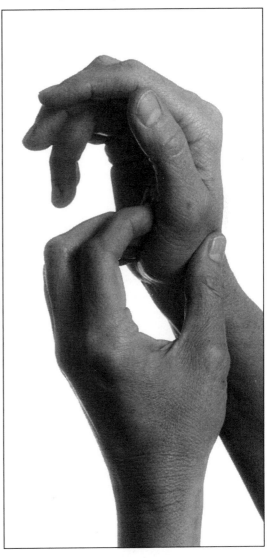

Suggestion: Try clamping into the base of the thumb and holding for 20 to 30 seconds with firm pressure. Use the thumb of your working hand to press around the base of your other thumbnail.

Thumbing the Palm and Wrist

Position: Place your thumb on the palm of the hand with your fingers on the back of the hand for support.

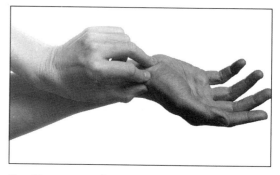

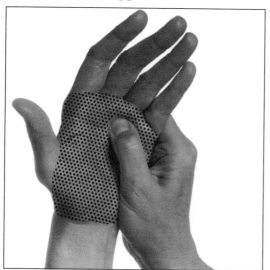

Directions:

1. Press into each point of the hollow areas in between the bones for five to ten seconds, using your thumb with your fingers directly in back of the thumb to increase the intensity of pressure being applied.
2. Make note of any painful points.

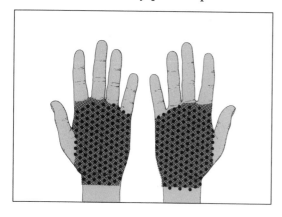

3. Return to these sore spots and hold them for a minute or two, with lighter, prolonged pressure. Hold the painful point steadily (without any motion, just light pressure) until you feel the pain subside.

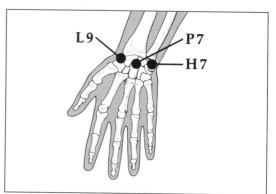

Suggestion: When you press into these palm points, slowly angle your pressure using a circular motion. The slower your rotations, the more beneficial the acupressure will be. Press into the wrist points, as illustrated, for 20 to 30 seconds each. These points are often very important for arthritis pain relief.

It is very helpful to gently rock the upper portion of the body forward as you exhale and apply the pressure. Inhale as you release the pressure, and let your chest and head rock backward.

Wrist Grasp

Position: Grasp the wrist with your working hand, keeping the palm of the working hand over the outside of the wrist.

Directions:
1. Squeeze the wrist for five seconds with your thumb and fingers wrapped around the inside of the wrist.
2. Repeat the squeeze several times in slightly different positions.
3. Apply light pressure around the wrist and slowly turn your working hand back and forth to gently wring the wrist.

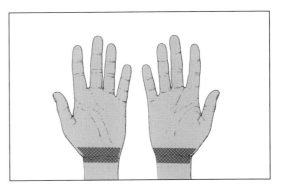

Suggestion: As you support the wrist, move your hand back and forth. Rotate your hand on your wrist a few times in one direction, and then the other, as you firmly hold the wrist with your working hand.

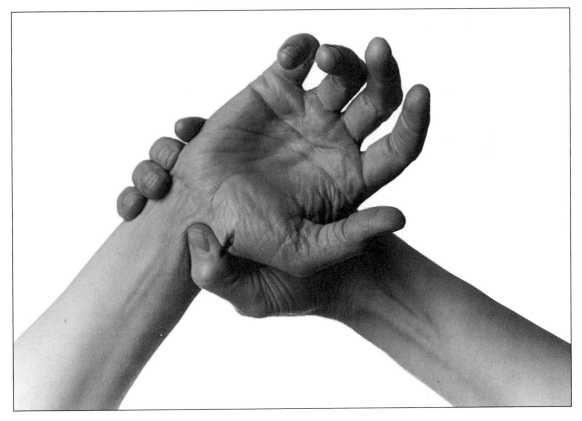

Wrist Points

Position: Grasp your wrist firmly. The palm of the hand being worked on can be facing up or down depending upon what is most comfortable.

Directions:
1. Bend your wrist to locate the joint at your wrist crease.
2. Firmly press into the hollow indentations in the joints for 30 to 60 seconds.
3. Gradually release your pressure. Slide your fingers around to find another indentation, and again hold for another minute.

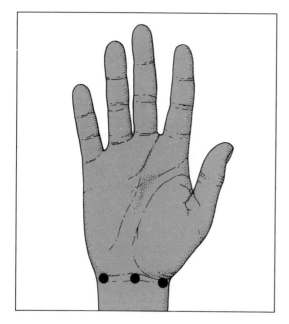

Suggestion: Slowly rotate your hand as you grasp your wrist for support. The combination of the rotation and the acupressure can strongly stimulate healing in the wrist and hand. If a wrist point is particularly sore, hold directly on the spot until the pain diminishes.

GOLF BALL HAND MASSAGE

Arthritis often leaves people with only partial use of their hands, making it difficult to apply the pressure needed in certain exercises. I have found that avocado pits and golf balls are both excellent tools for improving the condition of stiff, painful hands. The size and shape of a golf ball (or avocado pit or unshelled walnut) makes for a nice fit in the palm of the hand, enabling people with arthritis to apply a great deal of pressure without straining.

To effectively use a golf ball to massage your arthritic hands, you must learn to use the ball to obtain leverage and at the same time control the amount of pressure being applied. The next several pages will illustrate how to use a golf ball to stimulate various parts of the hand.

Try using your golf ball in your spare time while watching television, talking on the telephone, or whenever your hands are free. Experiment with different ways you can hold and move the ball to exercise your joints, release your tensions, and stimulate an increase in circulation.

Caution: When using the golf ball or avocado pit, always apply the pressure gradually. Jarring, rapid stimulation with these hard materials should be avoided to prevent an unnecessary injury or bruise.

Golf Ball Rolls: The Thumbs

Position: Wedge the golf ball between the index and middle fingers of your working hand. Place the ball on the palm side of your thumb, with the thumb of the working hand on top of the thumb being worked on.

Directions:

1. Slowly roll the ball up and down the length of your thumb. Move your other thumb directly behind the ball for support and leverage.

2. Position the ball directly on the most painful spots and hold with moderate, constant, steady pressure until you feel the pain or soreness subside.

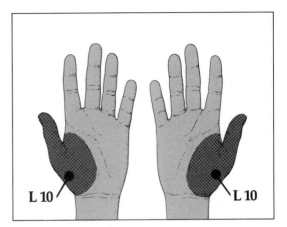

3. Reposition the golf ball on the center of the fleshy pad at the base of your thumb to press Point #2 for one minute.

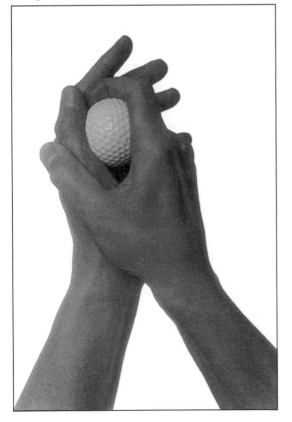

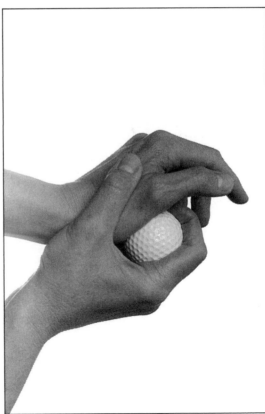

Golf Ball Rolls: Each Finger

Position: Use the palm of your working hand to hold the ball on the inside of one of your arthritic fingers. Wrap the fingers of your working hand around the outside of the finger being worked on, as illustrated.

Directions:

1. Slowly roll the golf ball up and down the length of each finger, resting the hand being treated on the top of your thigh for support.

2. Position the ball directly on your painful joints and hold with moderate, constant pressure until you feel the pain subside.

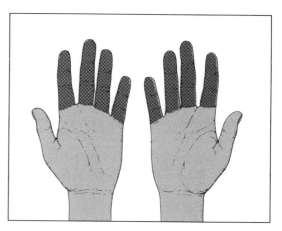

3. Roll each finger. Spend extra time working directly into your arthritic joints using prolonged, constant pressure.

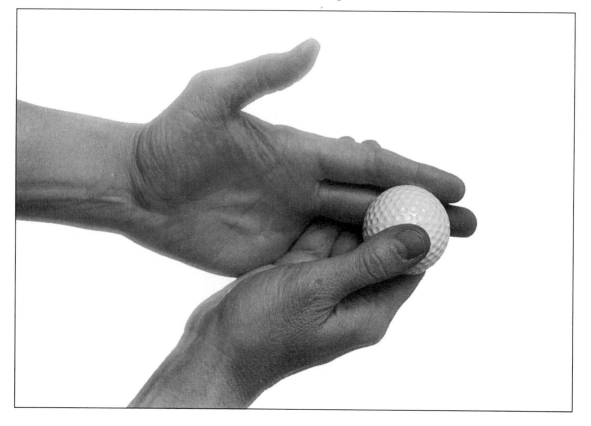

Golf Ball Rolling on the Anti-inflammatory Point[26]

Position: Place the golf ball between the thumb and index fingers on the outside of the hand being worked on. Hold the ball in place with the palm of your other hand.

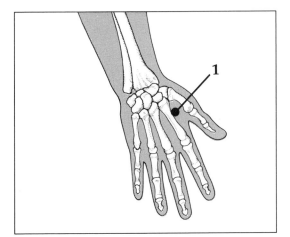

Directions:

1. Gently roll the ball in the webbing between your thumb and index finger for one minute.
2. Position the ball in the "V" where the thumb intersects with the index finger. Hold the ball steady for one minute using moderate pressure.
3. Move the ball a half inch toward the index fingernail (from the "V" juncture) and press directly on Point #1, as shown, for two or three minutes.

Suggestion: Repeat this two or three times daily (morning, afternoon, and evening) for best results to relieve your arthritic pain.

---

[26] The anti-inflammatory Point #1 is a general pain relief point, especially good for relieving arthritic pain, as well as constipation, toothaches, and most headaches. Please note that the anti-inflammatory point is *not* to be used during pregnancy.

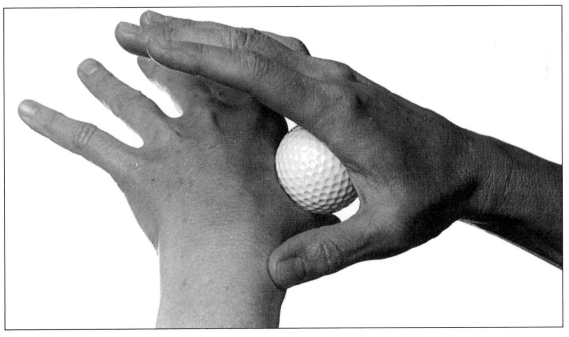

Golf Ball Presses in the Palms

Position: Place the ball between the palms of your open hands.

Directions:

1. Firmly clench the ball with both hands. Roll the ball gradually into different parts of the hand.
2. Position the golf ball on the most painful spots and hold with moderate, steady pressure until you feel the pain subside.
3. Reposition the ball in the center of the palm of your hand to press Point P 8 for one minute.

Suggestion: Try making one hand passive, the other active. Press into the passive hand as it relaxes. Then switch, making the active hand passive and vice versa.

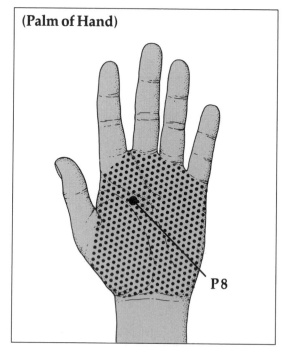

(Palm of Hand)

P 8

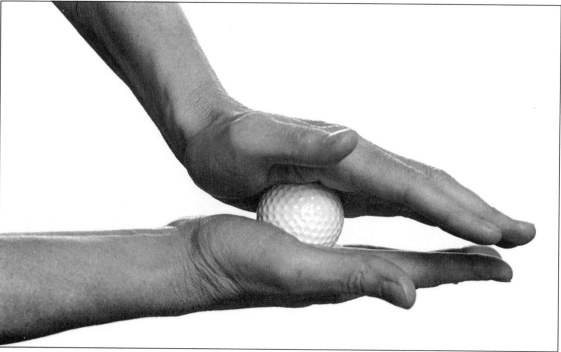

Golf Ball Clasp

Position: Interlace your fingers with your palms facing each other. Sandwich the golf ball between the heels of your two hands.

Directions:

1. Roll the ball slowly around all areas of your palms.
2. Roll the ball between your palms in small circular movements covering an area the size of a dime.
3. Make note of areas that feel sore or painful. Place the ball on those spots using only a mild amount of pressure. Hold the ball stationary in this position for a few minutes until the pain subsides.

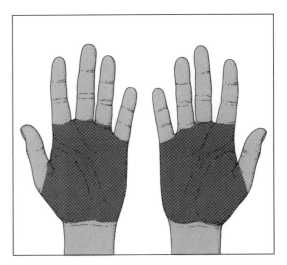

Suggestion: Place the golf ball between the inside center of your wrist crease and slowly roll the ball in small circles.

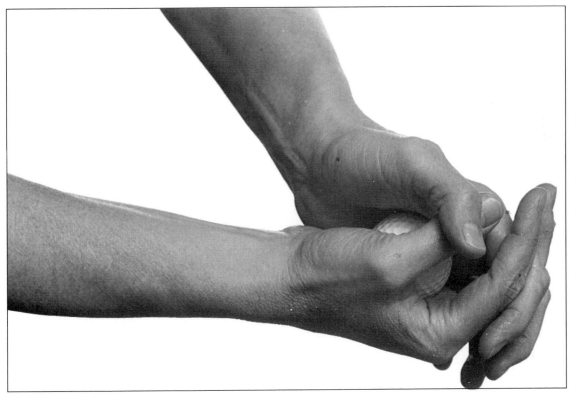

Golf Ball Finger Roll

Position: Place the golf ball in the palm of your cupped hand. Trap the ball between your thumb and fingers.

Directions:

1. Place one of your fingers (or thumb) between the golf ball and fingers of your working hand.
2. Slowly roll the ball over the finger, especially into the joints or stiff, painful areas.

Suggestion: Vary the amount of pressure you apply by tightening or loosening your grip. Hold the ball stationary (without any movement) directly on sore, painful spots, using light pressure for several minutes until the pain subsides.

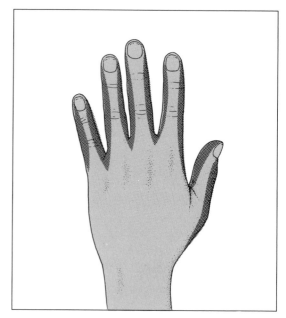

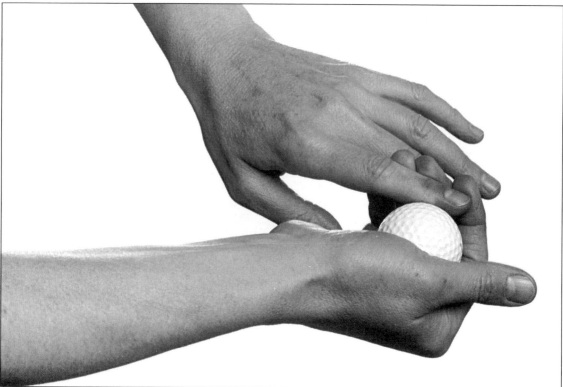

TECHNIQUES FOR HELPING OTHERS WITH HAND ARTHRITIS

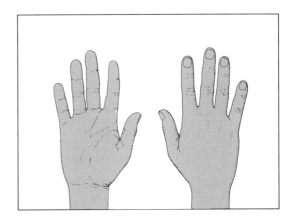

1. With both hands, firmly grasp and squeeze the hand with the receiving palm facing down. Use your whole hand to press from the wrist to the fingers. Knead the whole hand several times.
   Further Suggestion: As you slowly grasp the hand, gradually stretch it by spreading the bones apart.

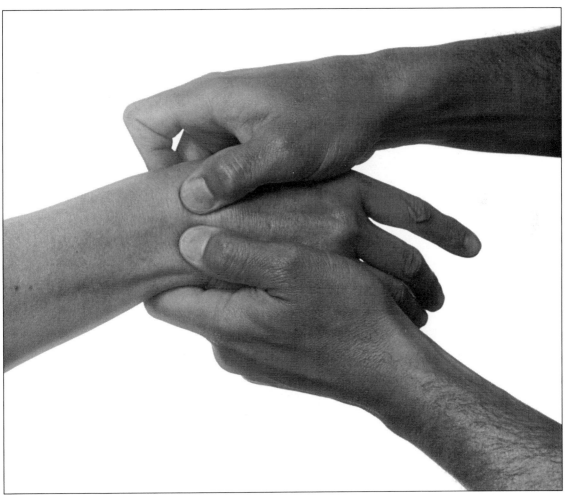

2. Press into the outside portions of the hand. Gradually apply firm pressure into the fleshy pads of the palm. Press into these pads as if you were modeling clay and kneading dough. *Further Suggestion:* Try kneading the hand firmly in very slow motion. Slow, conscious, graceful hand movements are extremely important in acupressure massage.

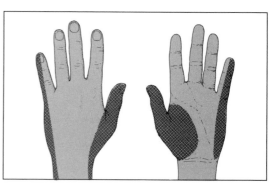

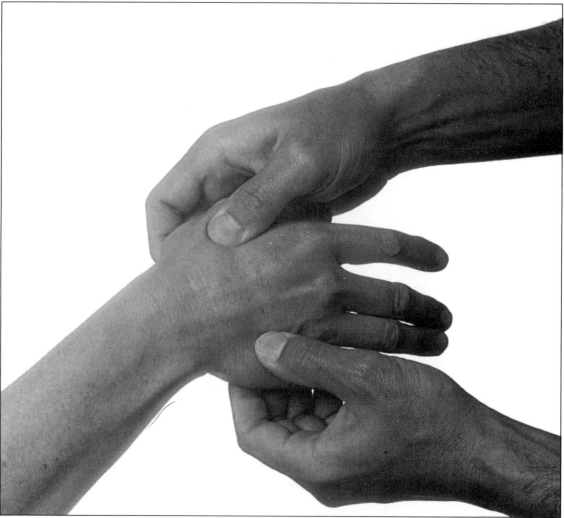

3. Press and roll each finger separately from the base to the tip. Pull each finger outward as you slide over it to put the joints in traction. Firmly squeeze the fingertip when you get to the base of the fingernail.
Further Suggestion: Rotate each finger in slow, small circles to relax the finger joints before you pull the finger outward, applying traction.

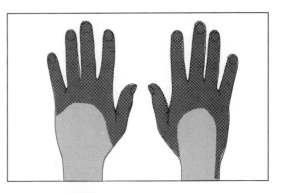

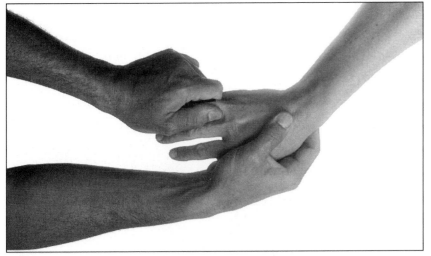

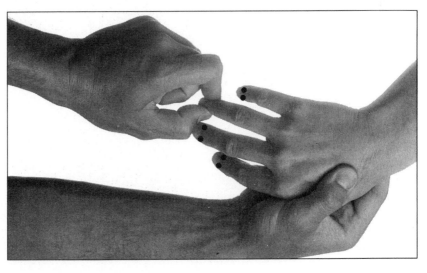

4. Massage the webbing between each of the fingers. These areas are important points for relieving arthritis in the fingers and hands.

Further Suggestion: After massaging the webbing between the fingers, return to each of these joints. This time, simply apply pressure in the hollow between the bones without any massage movement. Firmly hold each spot for at least a minute to help relieve pain.

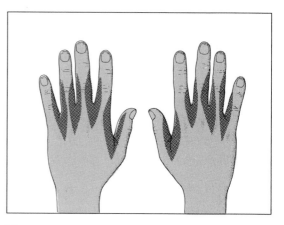

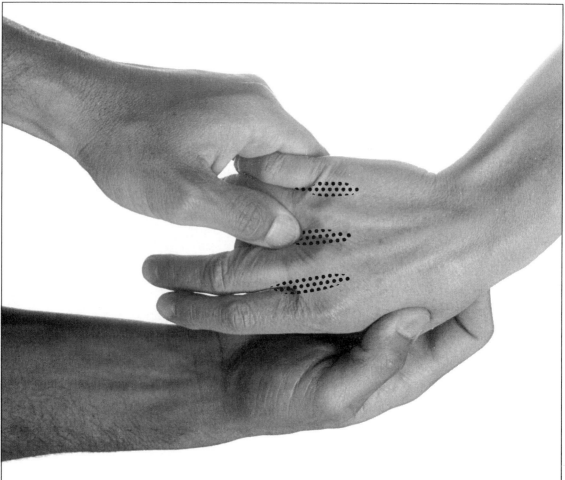

5. Thoroughly massage and press the webbing between the thumbs and index finger. With the palm of the recipient's hand facing down, press the outside of the hand with your thumb and use your fingers to press the palm.

Further Suggestion: As you press into the webbing between the thumb and index finger, angle the pressure toward and underneath the bone that attaches to the index finger.

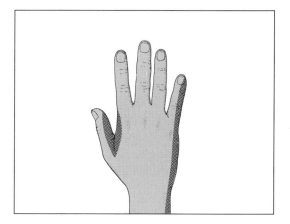

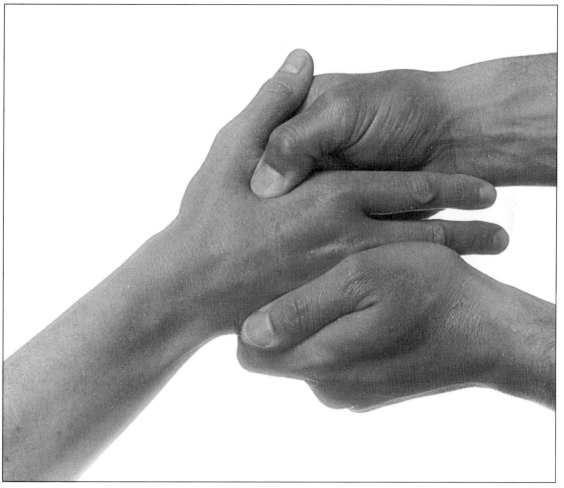

6. Press along the length of each finger.
Begin by firmly grasping the base of
the finger. Squeeze each segment of
the finger as you pull it outward, sliding toward the nail. Press and pull
out each finger in this way.
Further Suggestion: Press the base of
each fingernail using the thumb and
index finger of your other hand.
There are special acupressure points
at the side of each nail that are helpful
for relieving pain in the finger joints.
Press both sides of the base of the nail
for two or three minutes for pain
relief.

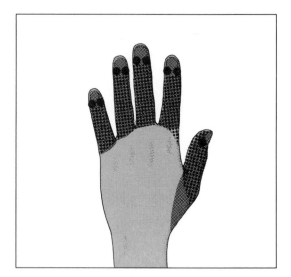

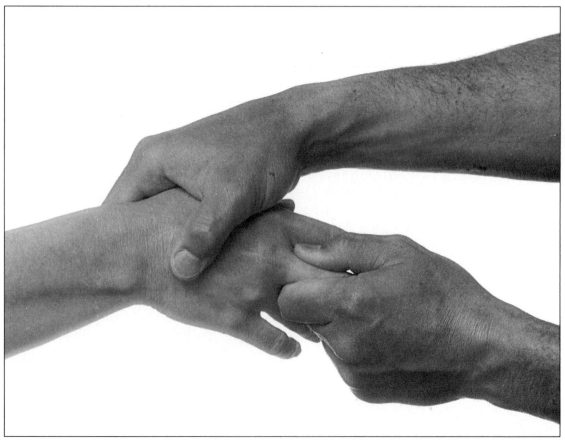

7. Turn the hand over. Press into the areas from the inside of the wrist to the center of the palm with your thumbs.
Further Suggestion: As you firmly press in, slowly rotate your thumbs to gently stimulate the area. If you find a sensitive or sore point, simply hold with light pressure for a couple of minutes to relieve the pain.

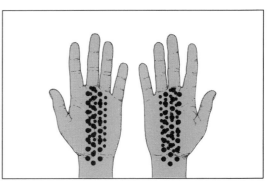

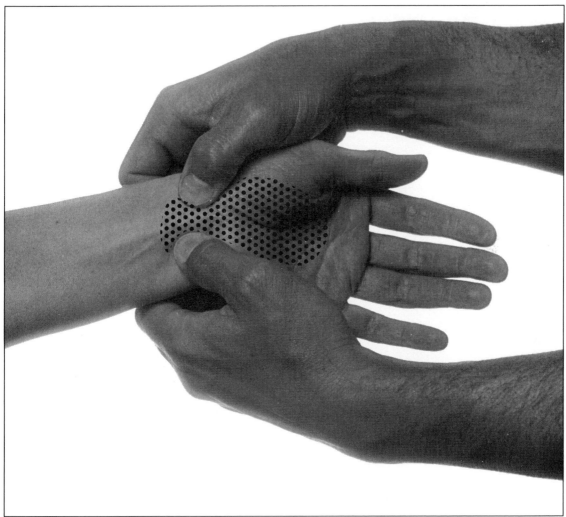

8. Press directly into the fleshy mound at the base of the thumb and the little finger.

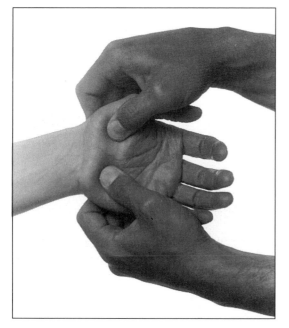

Further Suggestion: It is often effective to firmly knead these pads of the hand where tension often accumulates. This acupressure massage technique gently pinches and smoothes out tension in the mounds of the hands.

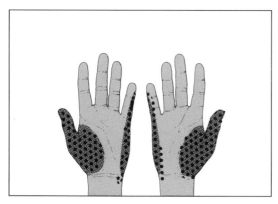

9. Use the knuckles of your fist to massage and press into the palm of the hand. Gradually press the palm for five to ten seconds. Slowly release the pressure and then press into a slightly different part of the hand.

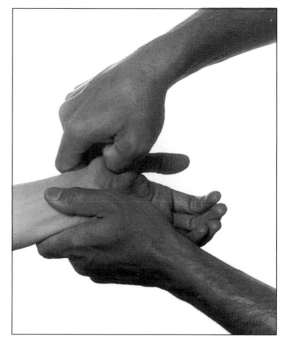

Further Suggestion: Smoothly rotate the direction of pressure being applied by your knuckles. Also try to slowly rub or roll your knuckles in the recipient's hand.

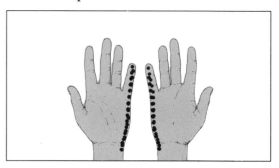

10. Use the first knuckle of your thumb to press various points on the hand. This can be a very powerful technique, so be careful not to press too hard.

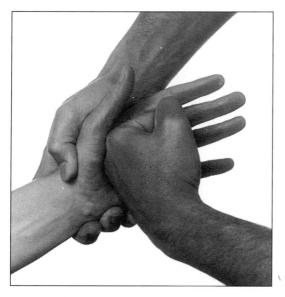

Further Suggestion: Use your index finger (of the same hand that is working) directly behind the pressure being applied with your thumb knuckle to grasp the area and give additional support.

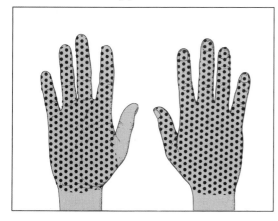

11. Bend the recipient's fingers into the palm. Enclose the hand in this position. Gradually squeeze it a few times.

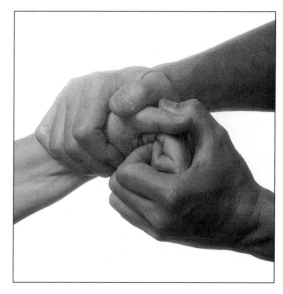

Further Suggestion: With your fingers in this position, rotate the recipient's hand on the wrist to firmly stretch the joints.

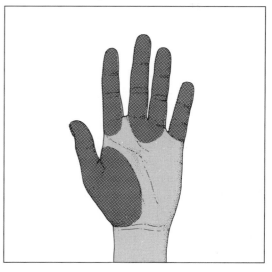

12. Interlace your fingers between the recipient's fingers. Slowly and firmly pull the fingers as you slide outward, giving the joints a gentle but firm traction.

Further Suggestion: Pull out each finger individually, and then again interlace your fingers between the recipient's fingers as you slowly pull the fingers outward to create firm traction.

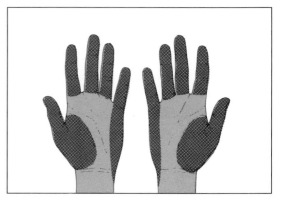

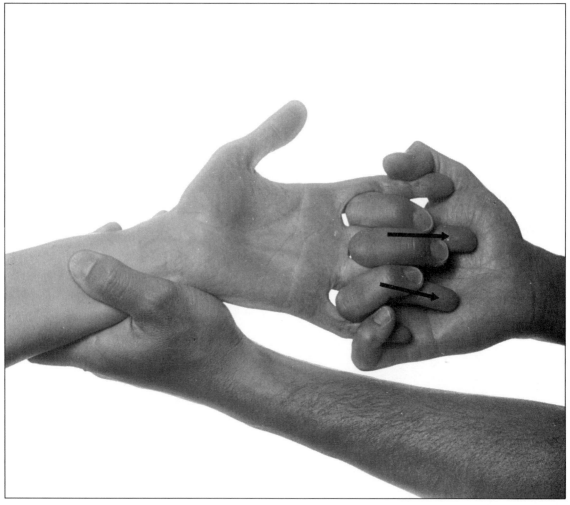

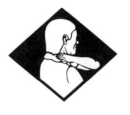

ARM AND
SHOULDER
PAIN

Arthritic pain in the shoulders usually begins with a dull aching that commonly escalates into severe shoulder pain. Certain movements of the arm or head can often aggravate this shoulder pain.

People with arthritis in their shoulders often have accumulated a great deal of chronic tension throughout the years. Modern lifestyles and stressful jobs create and reinforce shoulder tensions. Typing, working at a desk or over a machine or computer can cause shoulder tension. As your posture slumps, your breathing gets shallow. Tensions develop, and over the years inflammation can set into the joints. Truck drivers who hunch their shoulders as they hold the wheel develop these tensions. Anyone in competitive, stressful situations — whether an executive or a student — who does close work such as in electronics or graphic arts commonly suffers from shoulder pain from time to time.

One of my first patients, who lived in Los Angeles and owned a shoe company, had severe shoulder pain. Although he and his wife were intense and high-strung, they eventually let go of a lot of stressful obligations and responsibilities in their lives. While I was holding the acupressure points on his arthritic shoulders, he took a deep breath and exclaimed, "I feel as if you're pulling out large, rusty nails in my shoulders. The relief I feel is beyond words." Another patient of mine who had shoulder pain carried a mailbag on her shoulders for many years. She particularly complained of shoulder pain whenever she raised her arm. There was a click when she moved her arm back. Using acupressure Points #6, #7, and GB 21,[27] I helped her and many hundreds of people with these types of complaints, ranging from bursitis to shoulder pain due to an injury.

Arthritis in the shoulders, unless feverish, will respond well to hot compresses, along with stimulating the shoulder points and practicing the exercises that follow.

---

[27] These numbers refer to the acupuncture/acupressure point system of the body. You do not need to know any of these professional reference numbers to know how to practice the arthritis relief exercises and self-acupressure.

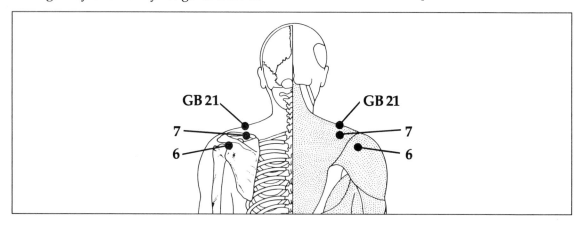

ARM AND SHOULDER PAIN
RELIEF POINTS

The following points are good for relieving pain and tension in the arms and shoulders. Apply one minute of firm pressure to each of the following points with your fingers curved in the shape of a hook.

GB 21 is the major point where shoulder tension collects. It is located on the top of the shoulder underneath the trapezius muscle. Traditionally, this point has been used for relieving stiff necks, rheumatism, and shoulder aches.

LI 14 is a special trigger point for relieving shoulder pain and chronic tension. Find a wiry band by rubbing your fingers over the bone on the outside of your arm. The point is at the bottom of the "V" of the muscle that covers the shoulder and upper arm. This point has been used for relieving toothaches, shoulder pain, arm aches, and stiff necks.

SI 11 is an excellent point for relieving tension and pain in the whole shoulder blade region. Feel for a large hollow area in the center of the shoulder blade. The point is usually very sensitive to strong finger pressure. This point has been used for neuralgia and pain in the scapula region and arm.

Point #5 helps to relieve arthritis in the elbow joint and is a trigger point for relieving arm and shoulder pain. It is also traditionally used to benefit the immune system and is especially good for relieving constipation.

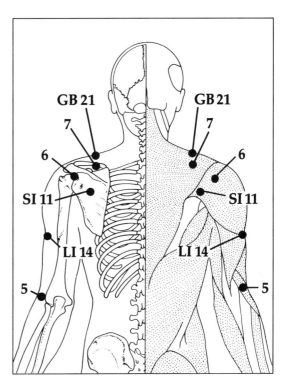

Point #6 is a key point for relieving arm and shoulder pain. It is located in the joint where the arm joins the back, directly between the top of the shoulder and the armpit crease. This acupressure point has also been used to relieve hypertension and shoulder bursitis.

Point #7 is an excellent point for relieving arthritic pain in the shoulders and arms. Feel for a marble of tension directly above the top inner point of the shoulder blade. This shoulder point has traditionally been used to reduce fevers and high blood pressure, and to relieve a stiff neck and nervous tension. A couple of minutes of firm pressure on Point #7 is helpful for increasing resistance to colds and flu.

SELF-ACUPRESSURE TECHNIQUES

Pounding Out Shoulder Tension

1. Make a relaxed fist with your right hand, keeping the wrist loose. Use the fist as a light hammer to pound your left shoulder.

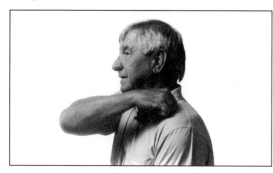

2. Maintaining this position, use the left hand on the right elbow to stretch the right arm backwards, pounding the back of the shoulders.
3. Continue the gentle pounding all around the arms toward the hand.

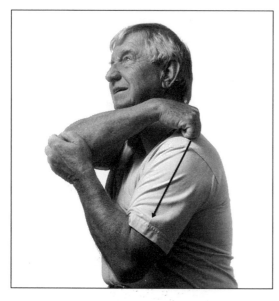

4. Now bring your hands to your knees. Sit up straight and close your eyes. Take a nice deep breath and feel the difference in your shoulders.
5. Then switch and work on your other shoulder and arm. Spend more time on the side that is tightest.

Arm Rub

Massage your arms thoroughly in a kneading fashion, progressing downward from your shoulders to your hands. Rub each arm for about five to ten seconds.

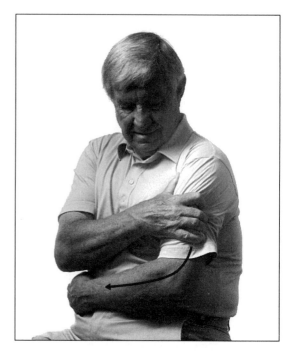

Arm and Shoulder Slap

Gently slap your arm to stimulate the circulation, moving from the top of the shoulder down to your hand. Repeat this twice on each side.

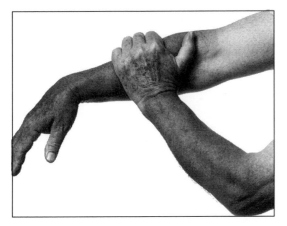

Forearm Squeeze

Knead the outer muscle of your forearm just below your elbow. Massage for five seconds, three times on each side.

Inner Elbow Massage

Rub your inner elbow in a circular motion with your fingertips. Massage for five seconds, three times on each side.

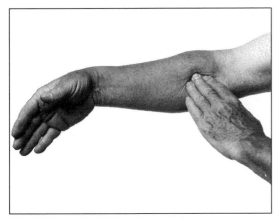

Shoulder Shrug

Shrug your shoulders six times up toward the ears. Inhale as the shoulders shrug up; exhale as they relax down.

SHOULDER MOBILITY— RANGE OF MOTION

The shoulder is the most mobile joint in the body. Pain, stiffness, and inflammation in the shoulder area (which includes the shoulder blade, upper arm, and collarbone) can severely limit the motions necessary for functioning in daily life.

The shoulder joint has tiny sacs of fluid that enable the muscles to move over each other smoothly. These bursas help to lubricate the joint to reduce friction. Shoulder pain and inflammation may be limiting your range of motion, thereby limiting functioning and circulation. Test yourself with the following arm movements to discover what your current range of motion is in your shoulder joints. Remember, avoid pain in any of these positions; move only as far as you can *comfortably* move.

Shoulder Range of Motion

1. While sitting or standing, raise your arms forward and up beyond your head. Then swing your arms back down and backward as far as you can without straining. Repeat this arm swing exercise two more times.

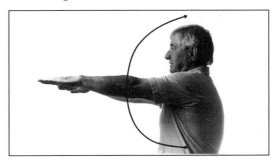

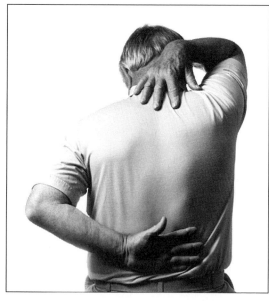

2. Try reaching over your shoulder and behind your back with the arms, as illustrated, attempting to touch the fingertips but without straining yourself. Reverse your arms and do the same stretch on the opposite side.

3. Raise your arms straight out at your sides with the palms facing up. Raise your arms until they touch your ears. If this is difficult, move slower and make the stretch gently. Repeat the exercise several more times, inhaling up and exhaling down.

Variation of Exercise 3: If you find it difficult to raise your arms, try lying in bed while raising your arms. Try this exercise with your elbows bent.

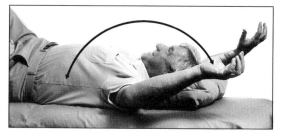

4. Place the palms of your hands against the back of your head. Inhale deeply as you slowly move your elbows out and backward. Exhale and relax, bringing your elbows together in front of you until they touch.

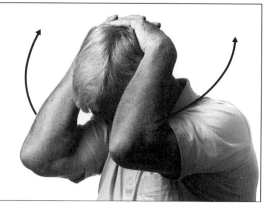

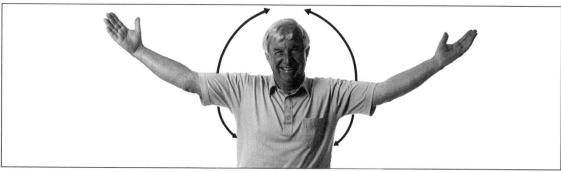

5. Then, try this circling motion with your entire arm, keeping the arm straight as you complete a wide circle. Do the movement with each arm.

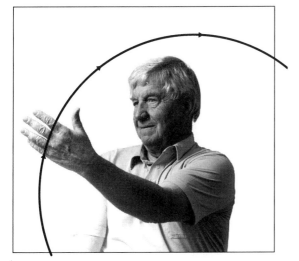

The following routine will both relax and strengthen the muscles in the shoulder area and help you increase your shoulder's flexibility. These exercises loosen the muscles to increase the circulation into arthritic or tight shoulders.

Pendulum Arm Swing

Directions:
1. Stand a foot away from the front of a chair.
2. Slowly bend forward, leaning the palm of your good, pain-free arm on the seat of the chair.
3. Let your other arm — the one giving you trouble — swing freely forward and backward.
4. Now swing the arm from side to side.
5. Finally, swing this arm in a small circle.

Suggestion: Try doing the same exercise while holding a weighted object in the hand of the swinging arm. Choose an object with a handle, like an iron or a gallon-size, half-full plastic water bottle. Follow the above instructions for the Pendulum Arm Swing while holding this object. If you practice this exercise regularly, using the water bottle, you can gradually increase the amount of water in the bottle. This will slowly increase the amount of traction you apply to your aching shoulder.

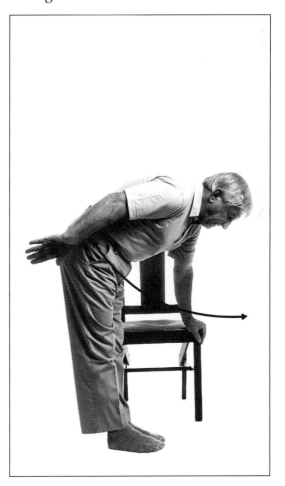

Swing Hands

This is an ancient exercise that has been handed down from generation to generation. Swing Hands enables the body to accumulate vital energy through the breath. It improves circulation, which energizes, awakens, and balances the body's energy, and contributes to a person's health and well-being.

The Chinese have documented numerous cases demonstrating that this exercise can also aid conditions such as insomnia, poor appetite, high blood pressure and heart trouble, eye problems, hemorrhoids, neurasthenia, and problems related to the liver, stomach, kidneys, and other internal organs.

Many of us live sedentary lives. We do not use our bodies enough to keep them vibrant and healthy. When we sit a lot, for example, the movement of the lungs is restricted, the digestive organs are compressed, and their proper functioning is thus hampered. Also, circulation is not stimulated the way it is by active movement, and it can become sluggish. Many health problems are either caused or worsened by an insufficient air supply and poor circulation.

The practice of Swing Hands can counteract these sedentary side effects. It is the simplest possible exercise besides walking, yet it moves and stretches the body, deepens the breathing, and improves circulation.

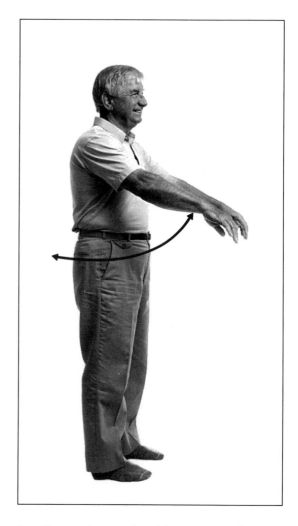

Directions:

1. Stand erect with your feet parallel and shoulder-width apart. Keep your knees slightly bent.

2. Grasp the earth with your toes by firmly curling them. If you wear shoes, your toes will grip the soles of the shoes.

3. Tighten your buttock muscles and contract your anus. This raises the rectum, which strengthens the reproductive and eliminatory systems. If you later notice that you have forgotten and have stopped doing the contraction, simply resume it.

4. Relax your upper body, including your chest, back, shoulders, arms, neck, head, face, and jaw.
5. Let your eyes look straight ahead, or close them if you prefer.
6. Swing your hands back and forth. As your arms come forward, they are parallel to the ground with the palms facing down. Vigorously swing them back to the limit of the arms' range of motion. This force leads directly to the easy forward swing, as action leads to reaction.

Suggestion: Count how many times you swing your hands. Start slowly with one hundred swings, if possible. You can gradually build up to two, four, five hundred, or even one thousand swings. For the greatest benefit, practice whenever you can, at various times during the day.

The feeling to cultivate is that of a light and relaxed upper body, with the lower portion of the body fully grounded and solid. Keep the back and head straight, as if they were being pulled up by a string. This will elongate the neck.

The shoulders, arms, hands, wrists, and elbows should be loose, moving easily. The chest should feel relaxed and open, allowing the breath to deepen naturally with the movement. The head, face, and jaw should be calm and relaxed. Make sure your knees remain bent throughout the exercise.

As you practice, be aware of your body, your breath, and your motion. Feel the aliveness and enjoy it!

Soaring Eagle

Directions:
1. Sit or stand with your arms relaxed at your sides and with your palms beside your thighs.

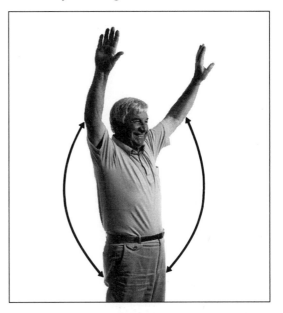

2. Inhale and raise your arms up and out to your sides until your arms are straight up above your shoulders.
3. Exhale as you gracefully let your arms float down to your sides, letting your shoulders relax.
4. Continue the exercise for one minute, inhaling as your arms soar up, and exhaling as they float down by your sides.

Suggestion: Tilt your head back as you raise your arms and inhale. Let your head fall forward and down as you exhale, allowing your neck to relax completely.

Shoulder Blade Press

Directions:
1. Stand with your feet shoulder-width apart.
2. Inhale as you interlace your fingers behind your back, with your palms facing each other.
3. Exhale as you bend forward and raise your arms up behind you.

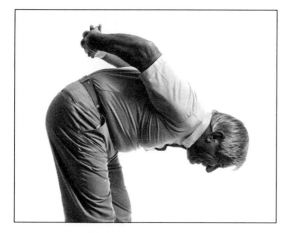

4. Inhale as you lower your arms and relax your shoulders, letting your arms dangle.
5. Continue the exercise a few more times. Then completely relax on your back or in a comfortable chair with your eyes closed for a few minutes to enable your body to assimilate the full benefits.

Suggestion: Once your arms are extended upward, flex your chest outward to further press your shoulder blades together.

Word of Caution: Patients with cardiovascular problems should practice this exercise carefully and/or consult a physician.

SHOULDER PAIN RELIEF EXERCISES

Rocking Between the Shoulder Blades

Directions:
1. Lie on your back with your legs bent and your feet flat on the floor.
2. Interlace your fingers behind your neck, lifting your head off the ground, with your elbows pointing upward.
3. Inhale and raise your pelvis upward, letting your head drop back down.

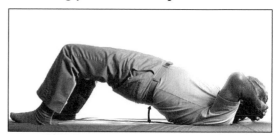

4. Rock back and forth on the upper part of your back by lifting your pelvis up high as your head comes down, and then raise your head upward as your pelvis lowers down. Continue this rocking movement several times with your eyes closed.

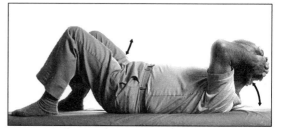

Suggestion: Make the movements rapid, and breathe deeply through your nose. After rocking between the shoulder blades for a minute, completely relax on your back with your eyes closed to maximize the benefits.

Shoulder Relief Bridge

Directions:

1. Lie on your back with your arms bent and your feet flat on the floor. You can keep your arms by your sides.
2. Inhale and raise your pelvis upward.

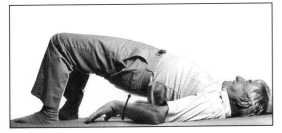

3. Hold this bridge position while you take a couple of long, slow, deep breaths.
4. Exhale and slowly come down.
5. Repeat the exercise several times.
6. Let yourself completely relax on your back with your legs bent and your eyes closed for a few minutes.

Suggestion: As you raise your pelvis up to a comfortable height, bring your hands up above your head with your arms bent, resting them on the floor above you. Push your feet against the floor, raising your pelvis a little higher (without straining yourself) to increase the pressure on your shoulders.

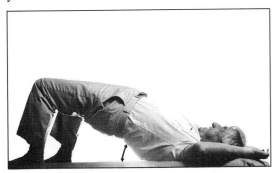

TECHNIQUES FOR HELPING OTHERS WITH SHOULDER PAIN

Shoulder Press

Recipient should be sitting on a low chair or stool, while you, the giver, stand close behind.

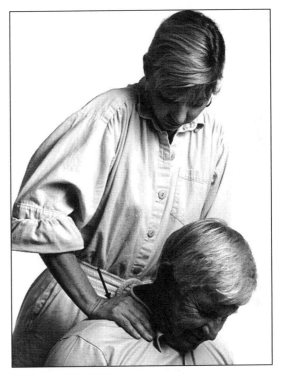

1. Place the heel of your hand on top of the recipient's shoulder bones with your fingertips resting on the upper part of the chest. Gradually lean your weight forward, slowly applying pressure to the top of the shoulders.

If the recipient feels pressure in his/her head, pressure was applied too fast and too hard. Concentrate on applying pressure gradually, moving into and out of the points slowly.

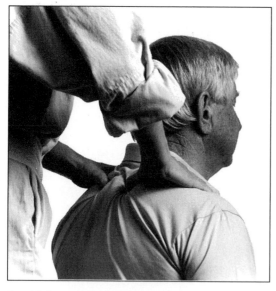

2. Take a step back from the recipient. In a standing position, place both hands on top of the shoulders. Use your thumbs to press down along the spine. Let your body lean into your thumbs to press into the large ropey muscles alongside the spine for five to ten seconds at a time. Continue down the upper back as illustrated. Keep your shoulders and arms relaxed.

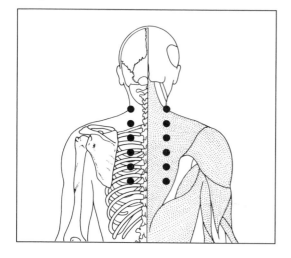

3. To more thoroughly cover the area in the illustration, use the second joint and knuckle of your index finger to press into the points. Gradually lean your weight toward the recipient as you apply pressure. Usually it takes about ten seconds to work on each of the points illustrated. If you feel a knot of tightness at any of these points, hold it firmly for about a minute to release this upper back tension.

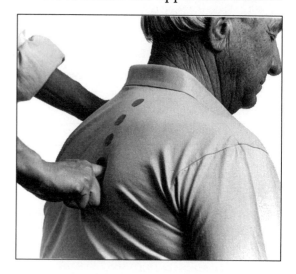

The thumb can be used to focus on the knots of tension that may accumulate underneath the shoulder blade. Support the left shoulder with your left hand while you work underneath the left shoulder blade. Ease the shoulder backward with your left hand, which will make the shoulder blade (scapula) protrude as you press on the back with your thumb. Switch hands to work on the other side.

You can also elevate the shoulder blade by applying pressure on the chest and upper arm. This will help stabilize the recipient as well.

Use the breath to help release tension and increase tolerance of pressure. The recipient should exhale as pressure is applied to the body and inhale as pressure is released. Maintain a rhythmic breathing pattern and coordinate it with your movements.

4. Place both of your hands on top of the recipient's shoulders with your fingers in front, thumbs on the back. Use your thumbs to press across the top of the shoulders (on the trapezius muscles). Press into the muscles gradually. Hold for five seconds at the depth of muscle tension. Slowly release the pressure. The three points illustrated on the top of the shoulder may be repeated three times for releasing shoulder tension.

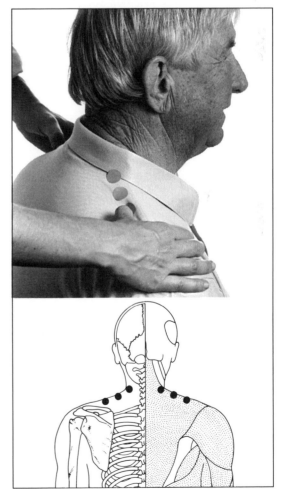

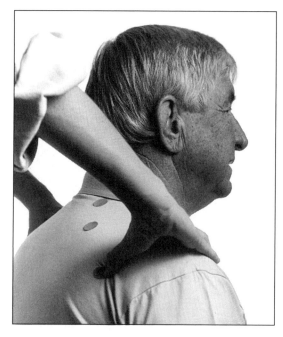

5. Bringing the thumbs back to the original position again, press into the points that curve diagonally below the armpit. Use your body weight, not your wrists, to apply the pressure.

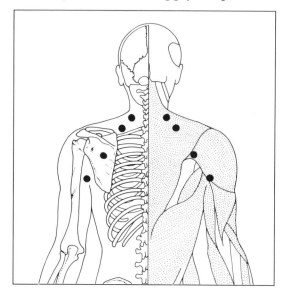

Lying Down Massage

Have the recipient lie comfortably on one side in a semifetal position on a padded surface. Use a pillow underneath his or her head to keep the vertebrae of the neck in line with the rest of the body.

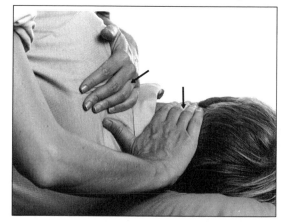

1. Use one hand to hold the side of the neck, and gradually pull back on the shoulder with your other hand. This will help stretch the muscles on the outside of the neck. Use your thumb to lightly press this muscle. Work from the top of this muscle, where it connects to the skull, down toward

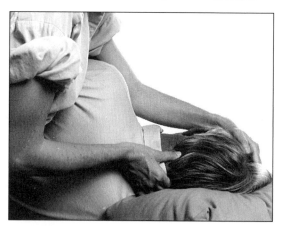

the shoulder. It is helpful to observe the recipient's facial expressions in order to obtain feedback about the amount of pressure being applied.

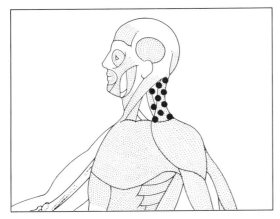

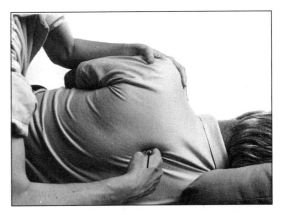

2. Kneel in back of the recipient. Firmly grasp one shoulder with your hands on both sides. Begin to move the shoulder up toward the ears and then pull it gently down. Flexibility will increase as the muscles relax. Start by moving the shoulder joint just a little. Increase the range of motion bit by bit as you feel the muscles begin to release.

3. The hand remaining closest to the recipient remains on the top of the shoulder for support. Use the thumb and bent index finger of your other hand to massage the shoulder blade. Slowly move the shoulder back with the hand that is on top so that the wing bone protrudes. Use the thumb and index finger to cover the length of the scapula. Moving the shoulder blade out will allow you to work underneath this bone, where muscular knots often accumulate.

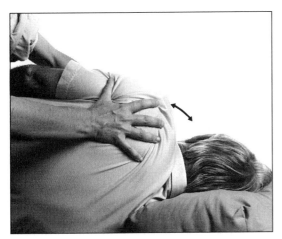

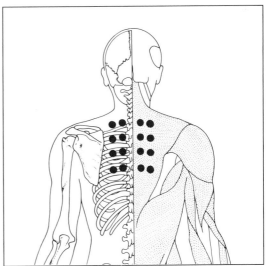

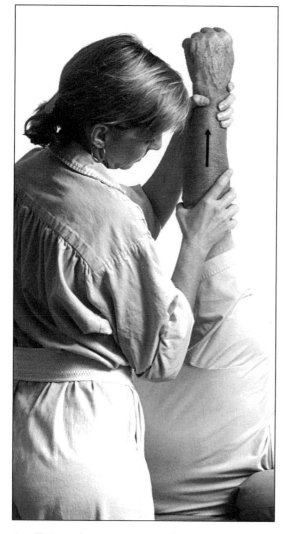

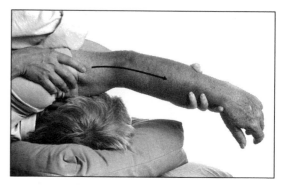

5. Grasp the recipient's upper wrist with your outer hand. Move the arm over the head, stretching it to the ear. Use the palm of your other hand to lean into the underside of the arm that is exposed. Work from the armpit up toward the elbow.

6. Return the arm to the recipient's side. Apply firm pressure with the palms of both hands to the outside of the arm down to the wrist. Keep your elbows straight. Gradually lean your body weight into the arm. Finish the arm by massaging the hand and pulling on each finger.

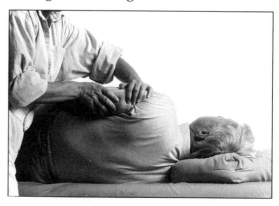

4. Bring the arm upward to a vertical position. Hold this arm up with both hands. Slowly pull upward on the arm, stretching the muscles that attach to the shoulder socket. Hold the extended arm up for a few seconds, and then carefully bring it down. Repeat this stretch a few times. Care should be given to the wrist as the arm is stretched.

Ask the recipient to turn over to work on the other side. Be sure to spend more time on the tightest or most painful side.

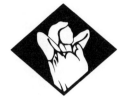

NECK PAIN

Arthritic pain in any part of the body, especially the extremities (hands, arms, feet, knees, legs, or hips) very often results in tightening of the neck muscles. The effect is pain and a decrease in the range of motion.[28]

Whenever arthritis settles in the neck, the corresponding neck muscles have difficulty supporting the weight of the head, which is usually fifteen to twenty pounds. Stress creates an additional burden on the neck muscles, and an unhealthy situation is set up where inflamed joints and tension breed more strain and often neck pain.

One of my clients had terrible neck pain for over ten years. Her doctors diagnosed her condition as cervical arthritis. She had pain that concentrated in her neck and radiated down her shoulders into her arms as well as into her head. Her pain was so severe that she had to be hospitalized and was put into traction. One of the top neurosurgeons in the country gave her a neck-waist brace to help control her pain. This brace stabilized her body, but she was anxious to make more progress. After a couple of acupressure sessions, she had such substantial relief that she no longer needed the brace at all.

Another elderly client of mine who suffered from severe neck pain had limited mobility in her neck as well. After the initial injury, she spent some time in traction at home, and her neck became extremely tight and painful. She proceeded to try numerous approaches —

including physical therapy, daily medication, biofeedback — none of which seemed to give her any relief from her pain or to increase her range of motion. Feldenkrais movement therapy did help her to some degree, but she still felt she could be making more progress.

After her first acupressure session, she reported that she had more relief from the acupressure than from any of the other methods she had tried in the past eighteen years. She not only had relief from the discomfort, but also had a feeling of stability in her neck. She felt more aligned and in balance, and had a range of motion that she hadn't had for years.

Once she began to learn acupressure, she found she was able to help herself as well. The acupressure points under the base of the skull made a significant difference in relieving her pain and erasing what she called her "hot spots." Whenever it becomes difficult for her to turn her neck and the pain begins to creep up on her, she continues to practice these self-acupressure techniques.

SELF-HELP FOR THE NECK

There are many self-help techniques for relieving the chronic neck tension that often occurs from tensing against arthritic pain. I have found that a combination of Acu-Yoga (using posture to press the acupressure points for self-treatment), hot compresses, deep breathing, and acupressure are particularly effective. First, apply the hot compresses to your shoulders and neck until the skin becomes pink,

---

[28] Semyon Krewer, *The Arthritis Exercise Book*, Simon & Schuster, 1981.

indicating an increase in circulation. Ginger compresses are highly effective for relaxing the muscles in this area. [29]

If the compresses are inconvenient or unavailable, do the Dry Wash described below. After doing the Dry Wash Facial Massage or applying the hot compresses, rotate your head very slowly five times in one direction and then the other. Keep your eyes closed and breathe deeply as you do this exercise. This will help to elongate the neck and naturally reposition the vertebrae in the cervical region.

Dry Wash Facial Massage

1. Rub your hands together, creating a heat.
2. Immediately afterwards, thoroughly massage your face and neck with the palms of your hands.

Benefits: A daily dry wash cleans the pores, restoring tone and luster to the skin. This warming massage is helpful for acne and stiff necks.

---

[29] See page 210 for the directions to make ginger compresses.

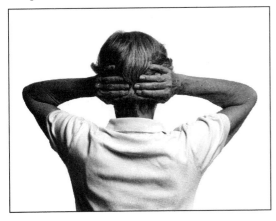

Beating the Heavenly Drum

This exercise stimulates the acupressure points under the base of the skull.

1. Sitting comfortably, place your middle fingers on the base of your skull, and cross the index fingers over the middle fingers.
2. Cover your ears firmly with the palms of your hands.
3. Snap the index fingers against the middle fingers on the occipital ridge for approximately one minute. Listen to this drumlike sound in your inner ear.

Benefits: Relieves arthritic neck pain, headaches, neck tension, burnout, eyestrain, and dizziness.

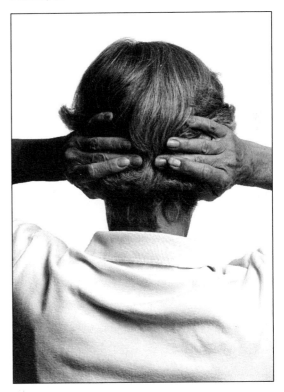

Look Behind

1. Stand with your arms crossed in front of your upper chest. Keep the chin tucked into the hollow of the throat, stretching the back of the neck.

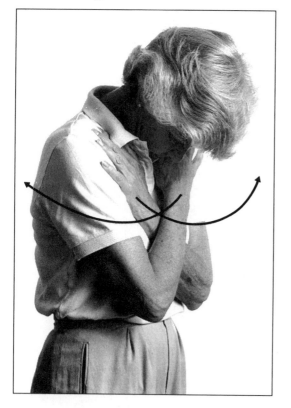

2. Inhale deeply, open your arms to a 45-degree angle from the sides of your body, and turn your head toward the left, looking as far behind you as possible. Pull your arms back, arching the chest up and out. You will feel the stretch in your arms, wrists, neck, and also your eyes as you look behind.
3. Exhale, returning your head and arms forward.

4. Repeat the same movement, turning to the right side. Alternate sides, practicing the movement six times in all.

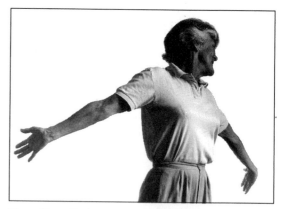

Benefits: Relieves arthritic neck and shoulders, prevents stiff necks, hunch back, and pain in the upper back. This exercise also increases your resistance and expands the capacity of the lungs.

Neck Stretches

1. Place your left hand over the top of your head on your right side. Pull your head to the left, stretching the right side of your neck. Reverse sides and repeat several times.

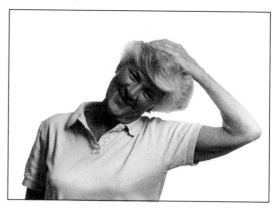

2. Interlace your fingers behind your neck. Inhale as you tilt your head back and stretch your elbows up and backward.

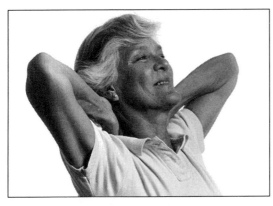

3. Exhale, letting your head and elbows slowly relax forward. Continue to inhale up and exhale down. Repeat steps 2 and 3 at least six more times.

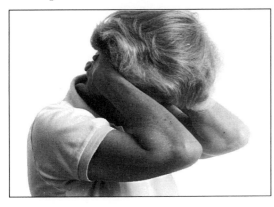

Benefits: Relieves shoulder and neck arthritic pains, stiff necks, and tightness in the shoulders and helps to improve the overall circulation. Meditate or relax on your back with your eyes closed for at least a few minutes after practicing these neck stretches to assimilate the benefits of these exercises.

NECK POINTS

The following acupressure points are good for relieving pain and tension in the neck. Apply one minute of firm pressure to each of the following points as shown in the photographs. Point #8 is located

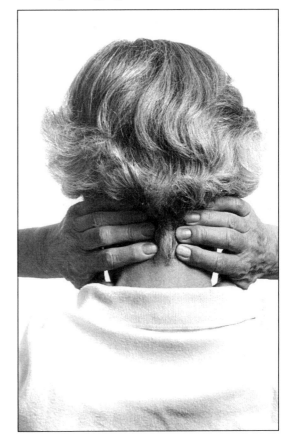

on the upper portion of the neck, approximately one thumb's width from the spine. To find this point, start from the outside of the two large ropey muscles that run parallel to the spine and press in very gradually one-half inch below the base of the skull. If you have severe neck tension in this area, you may also find small hard lumps about the size of a pea. Hold the tightest point on your neck for three minutes as you breathe deeply.

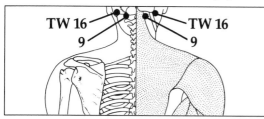

Benefits: Relieves arthritic stiffness, rigidity, pain in the neck and back, neck spasms, throat spasms, nervous system disorders, and is especially useful in times of stress and trauma.

Point #9 is located just below the base of the skull, in a hollow between two muscles.

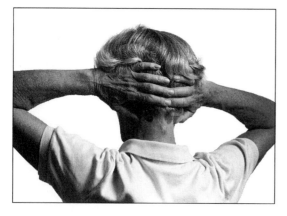

Benefits: Relieves neck arthritis, as well as headaches, back pain, stiff neck, insomnia, nervousness, mental pressures, and trauma.

TW 16[30] is located underneath the outside base of the skull, behind the earlobe.

Benefits: Relieves arthritic shoulder pain, backaches, arm pain, stiff neck, eye pain, earaches and pressure, and facial swelling.

Neck Press

1. Lie on your back. Clasp your hands together behind your neck.
2. Exhale and slowly pull the head up, using your arm muscles. The heels of the palms should be firmly pressing the sides of your neck.

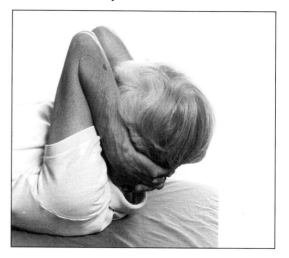

3. Breathe deeply, keeping your head up and your elbows as close together as possible for one minute.
4. Inhale deeply and hold for a count of ten, stretching your neck further.
5. Exhale and slowly lower the head to the floor. Relax with your arms by your sides, eyes closed, and discover the benefits.

Benefits: Relieves arthritis, sore throat, acne, stiff neck, thyroid irregularities, mental disorders, speech problems, or general pain.

---

[30] I'd like to point out once again that these letters and numbers refer to the acupuncture/acupressure point system. You do not need to know any of these reference numbers to practice the Arthritis Relief Program.

Rolling the Head

1. Lie on your back with your arms and legs comfortably relaxed.
2. Let your head slowly roll from side to side. Close your eyes and feel your neck relax as your head gently moves.

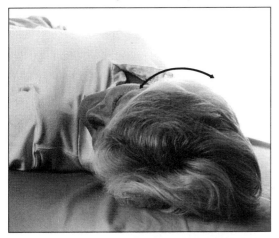

3. Let your breath be long and deep.
4. Continue the subtle movement until you can completely relax your neck.
5. Finish with your head straight in line with the spinal column. Relax with your hands by your sides for another few minutes.

Benefits: Eases arthritic pain and stiffness, balances repressed anger, nervous disabilities, insomnia, headaches, neck pain, and depression. For adequate self-treatment, continue practicing the neck exercises in this section as a routine for six weeks, two or three times daily.

Caution: If you have had a recent whiplash, wait until most of the inflammation from the neck injury diminishes before you begin to practice these self-help techniques, or consult with your physical therapist or doctor.

TECHNIQUES FOR HELPING OTHERS WITH NECK PAIN

1. Begin by having the recipient sit comfortably on a stool or pillow. Stand close behind the recipient's back. Place the palm of your hands close to the neck over the top of the shoulders.

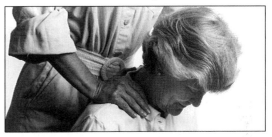

Slowly lean your body weight into the shoulder tension (the trapezius muscle) with the heel of your hands for about 30 seconds. Slowly release the pressure. Repeat this a few more times, moving your hands over slightly different spots where there is muscular tension.

2. Interlace your fingers. Place the palms of your hands on either side of the recipient's neck. Press firmly into the neck muscles for one minute.

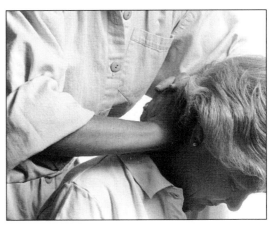

3. Place your right hand under the base of the skull. Tilt the head back with your left palm supporting the forehead. Press the points underneath the base of the skull with your right hand as you lift the head upward for approximately 30 seconds. Then very gradually release the pressure.

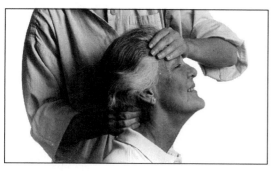

4. Visually divide the length of the neck into three sections: upper, middle, and lower. Sitting toward the left side of the recipient, place your right hand on the neck with the thumb on the left side and fingers on the right side. Begin with the upper portion of the neck. Slowly bring your fingers together like a vise until your fingertips firmly meet the level of muscular tension. Hold this level for a few seconds and then slowly release the pressure. Slide your hands down, covering all parts of the neck. Repeat this three times for people with neck tension. If you are larger than the recipient, then caution should be taken to avoid extreme pressure on the jugular vein.

    Encourage the recipient to breathe into any tense areas to relax the muscles.

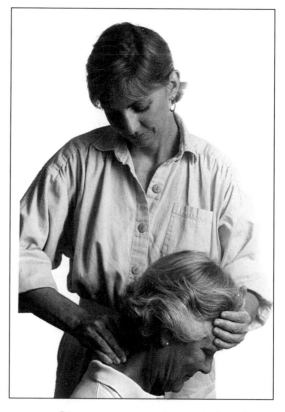

Give support to the recipient by holding the forehead as your other hand works on the neck.

5. Stay on the left side of the recipient. Place your right thumb into the hollow at the base of the skull. Support the forehead with your left hand.

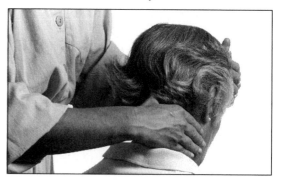

Rotate the thumb clockwise as you press into the hollow and up underneath the base of the skull. Gradually begin to move the head around. Securely support the head with both hands in this position, encouraging the recipient's neck muscles to relax as the head slowly moves in a wide circular motion.

6. Place your hand on the top of the shoulder. Cross the index finger over the middle finger snugly against the left side of the neck. Use your other hand to stretch the neck sideways to the left, as shown. Then place the opposite hand on the right side and ease the head gradually to the right. This movement helps to stretch out chronic neck tension that reinforces arthritic aches and pains in the shoulders and neck. It also works on the

large intestine and gall bladder meridians, which can help prevent as well as relieve headaches, including migraine headaches. Ease the head gradually to both sides.

7. Next, place the back of your fist on the shoulder, close against the neck. Hold the forehead with your other hand, bending the recipient's head back toward the fist. Maintain this

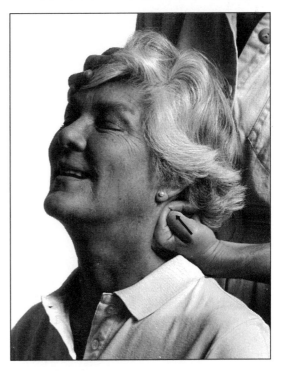

position, as shown, for approximately ten seconds. Gradually release the pressure and repeat the move on the other side. This, along with the next technique, is helpful for migraine headaches. Make sure to apply the pressure gradually. It should feel good, somewhere between pain and pleasure.

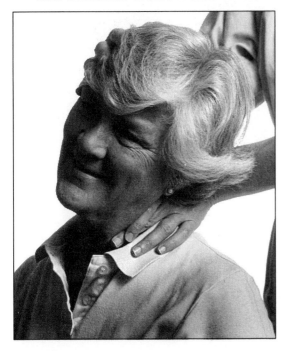

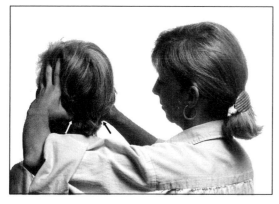

8. Place your thumbs under the base of the skull. Tilt the recipient's head back a little while you firmly stretch the head straight up, pressing Point #9 underneath the base of the skull.

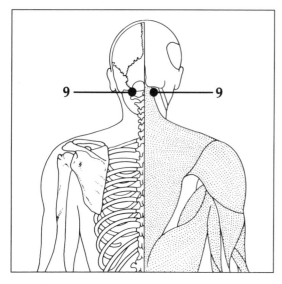

Blockage at this point is many times the source of headaches. It is sometimes called the "Gates of Consciousness" since it helps regulate the sensorial and neurological activities of the brain. Have the recipient inhale as you elevate and exhale as you release.

Cradling the Head

1. Have the recipient lie down on his or her back. Sit just behind the top of the head, and gently bring the hair out from under the neck. Sensitively knead the muscles at the back of the neck, using your thumb and fingers to squeeze out the tension. This acupressure massage technique is most effective when done very slowly.

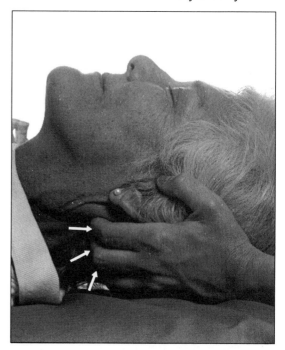

2. Hold the head in your palms, with the backs of your hands resting on the ground. Support the whole skull with your fingers curved, gradually pulling it outward. Slowly rake the skull, gliding your fingertips over the head. Imagine that the contact of your hands is a communication of love and support.

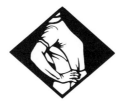

BACK PAIN

Back problems are one of the most common ailments in our society. Almost everyone has experienced stiffness, tension, or pain in some part of the back, and some people suffer for years. Arthritics are even more vulnerable to the negative effects of poor posture, lack of flexibility, and stress, all of which can produce back pain and weakness.

It is especially important to strengthen the muscles surrounding the spine so that the vertebrae are stabilized and discs stay in place. If those muscles are weak, the sciatic nerve can be damaged, causing severe pain and even numbness along the buttocks and legs.

Acu-Yoga, the combination of acupressure point stimulation with gentle yoga stretching exercises, effectively releases tension and restores the natural harmony of the body. Working to improve your posture, strengthen and relax your back muscles, and increase the flexibility in your spine can help tremendously in reducing back discomfort and will ultimately have a beneficial effect on your general health as well.

A Word of Caution: Anyone with a back problem should be sure to practice Acu-Yoga carefully and to move slowly and gently into and out of the postures. No exercise should be practiced in a jolting or jarring fashion. No exercise should be pushed beyond your limit. STRETCH — DON'T STRAIN! If you still have doubts, consult your doctor, chiropractor, or physical therapist before you try these exercises — especially if you have had back surgery or severe disc problems.

ACU-YOGA SELF-TREATMENT PLAN

1. Choose three or four exercises that relate to your problem, using the index or the chapter headings in this section.
2. Practice these exercises two or three times a day for one week. Gradually increase the time spent in each posture.
3. After the exercises, cover yourself with a blanket and lie on your back with eyes closed. Take several slow, deep breaths and allow yourself to completely relax for ten minutes.

THE UPPER BACK

Self-Help

The upper back is one of the most difficult areas to reach on yourself in order to apply finger pressure. For self-care, try placing a tennis ball or a small, hard ball such as a racquetball beneath the tender areas as you lie on your back and breathe deeply.

You can also ask a friend to gradually press directly into any "knots" in your upper back. These knotted areas are often acupressure points and may be quite tender at first touch. Maintain a firm but gentle pressure on these points for one to five minutes or until any soreness diminishes and the "knots" begin to relax and disappear.

The following acupressure points on the hands and arms, held with the upper back points, often help facilitate this release.

Trigger Points

Point #1 is used to relieve arthritis in the back and neck, headaches, migraines, toothaches, constipation, and neuralgia.

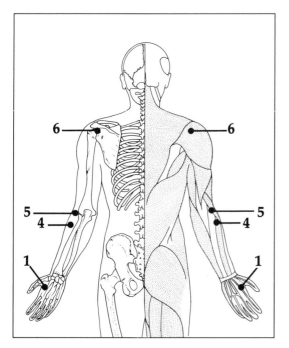

Point #4 is used for muscular spasms in the arm or upper back, indigestion, swollen or stiff neck, and poor circulation.
Point #5 helps to relieve constipation, depression, upper back pain and brachial or intercostal neuralgia.
Point #6[31] releases the shoulder girdle and upper back area. (Traditionally, this point has been used for hypertension, insomnia, anxiety, nervousness, arm pain or numbness, and cold hands.)

---

[31] These point numbers are used for reference only. You do not need to know them to practice the Arthritis Relief exercises and self-acupressure.

UPPER BACK EXERCISES

Practice the following Acu-Yoga exercises and/or utilize tennis balls to apply pressure between your shoulder blades. Allow two minutes for each exercise and three minutes with the tennis balls. Then spend about ten minutes relaxing your back and breathing deeply.

Upper Back Opener

Stand with your feet about shoulder-width apart. Inhale as you interlace your fingers together behind you. Exhale as you bend forward and raise your arms

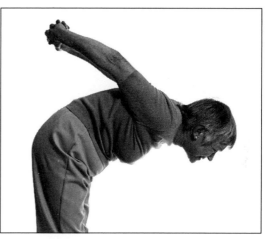

up behind you. Stretch your arms upward, moving your shoulder blades toward one another. Inhale as you lower your arms and return to a straight, standing position. Continue the exercise several times.
Benefits: This is an excellent exercise for arthritis in the upper back, as well as for relief of hypertension, upper back and shoulder tension, arm problems, cold hands, anxiety and insomnia.

Pelvic Lift

Lie on your back with your legs bent and your feet flat on the floor. Inhale and raise your pelvis upward. Exhale and slowly come down. Repeat the exercise several times.

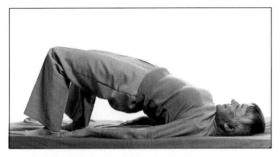

Benefits: This Acu-Yoga exercise not only benefits the spine and the pelvic region, it also effectively releases muscular tension in the shoulders.

THE LOWER BACK

Although the majority of lower back problems are directly related to stress, poor posture, accidents or weak musculature in the abdominal region, traditional Chinese medicine teaches that pain or tensions in the lower back are associated with the bladder, kidneys, and reproductive system.

The kidneys are considered the storage tanks of the body, gathering surplus energy and storing it to be used when needed. When the kidneys have an abundance of this reserve energy, the lower back will be strong and flexible. However, deficiency or weakness in the kidneys — brought on by "running on nervous energy," eating too much salt, drinking too much liquid or not drinking enough, excessive sexual activity or excessive fear — can cause problems in the lower back.

The following Acu-Yoga exercises relieve tension and strengthen the lower back.

Self-Acupressure Massage

In a standing position or sitting on the edge of a chair, place your fists on both sides of the lower back and gently but briskly rub 100 to 200 times. Continue to rub from your lower back to the buttocks with the backs of your hands until your lower back feels warm. Practice this self-acupressure massage technique two or three times daily.

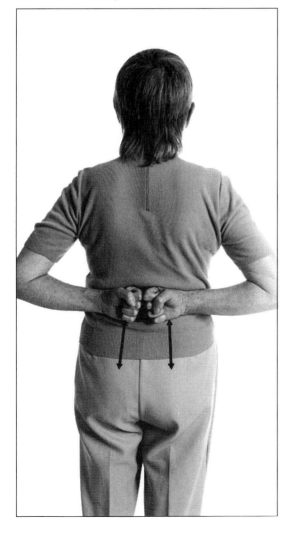

Hip Rotations

Move your hips around in a full circle. Rotate your pelvis several times in one direction and then the other. Breathe deeply and enjoy the movement.
Benefits: This exercise can prevent many lower back problems. The movement stretches the muscles in the pelvis and lower back. People who have lower back problems with accompanying tension or stiffness should do the exercise several times a day. Make the movements slow and easy, without pushing yourself.

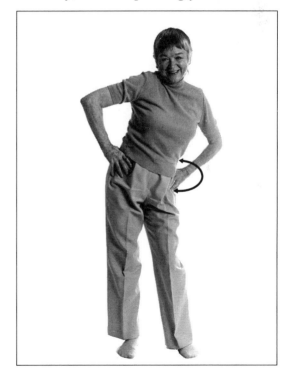

A Word of Caution: If you have acute pain from an accident or injury, hip rotations may not be advisable. Consult a doctor or physical therapist with any individual questions about these exercises.

Spinal Flex

The following exercise stimulates the spinal nerve cord, which branches out and down from the brain. This nerve cord is protected in the body vertebrae by three layers of membranes and the cerebrospinal fluid that flows between them and also through the brain itself. The following exercise flexes and extends the spine back and forth, gently stretching the spinal muscles that hold the vertebrae in place. This enables the cerebrospinal fluid to circulate freely and improves the condition of the spine and of the back muscles.

1. Sit comfortably in a chair.

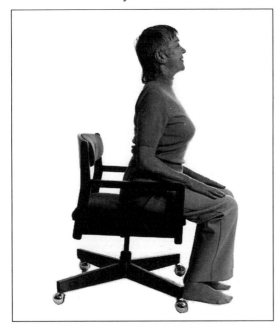

2. Place your palms on your thighs, with your spine straight.
3. Inhale and arch your spine, gently but firmly pushing your chest outward.

4. Exhale and let your spine slump back into a round curve. This stretches the spine in the opposite direction. Let your head relax downward with each exhalation.

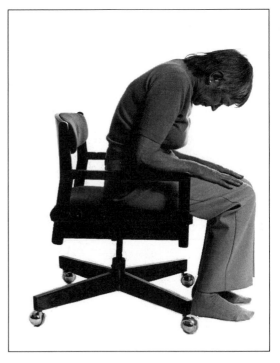

5. Continue for one minute. Begin slowly and gradually, feeling the motion and stretch in your back. Gradually increase speed as your back loosens up. Breathe with each movement, inhaling as the chest pushes outward, and exhaling as you slump back and down.
6. Completely relax on your back for a few minutes.

Benefits: This exercise relieves spinal stiffness, back aches and pains, indigestion, nervous disorders, postural problems, and cold feet.

Lower Back Bends

1. Stand with your legs one foot apart and your feet facing straight ahead.
2. Inhale, bringing your hands to your waist with your thumbs pressing your lower back.
3. Exhale as you gently bend back, and inhale again as you straighten up.

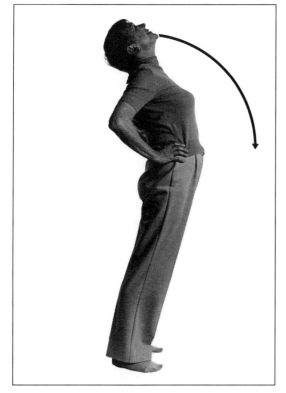

Exhale as you let the weight of your upper body bring you forward with your head near your knees. Inhale up, exhale down.
4. Repeat the exercise five times.
Benefits: This movement aids in the flexibility of the spine and benefits the kidneys. It is excellent for relieving fatigue.

Cat Cow

1. Kneel on all fours.
2. Inhale as the head goes back and you arch the spine.

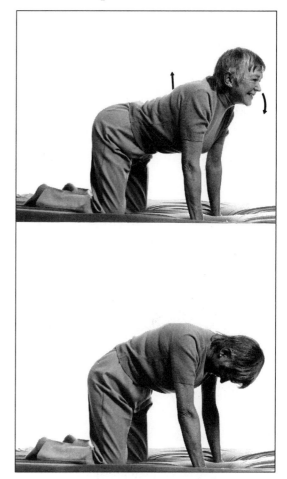

3. Exhale as the head comes down and the spine curves up. Make the movement rhythmic.
Benefits: This flexibility exercise helps to relieve arthritic pain in the middle and lower regions of the spine as well as strengthen the lower back and the reproductive organs.

Knees to the Chest

This is one of the best exercises to prevent and relieve lower backaches. As you bring your knees in toward the chest, the mid-lower back flattens to the floor, pressing on the lower back points that correspond to and benefit the kidneys, the intestines, and the digestive system.

1. Lie on your back. Comfortably tilt your head back.
2. On an exhalation, bring your knees up to your chest, using your hands to hold Spleen 9 (Sp 9), on the inside of the leg just underneath the knee bone.
3. Use your arm muscles to help bring your knees to your chest.

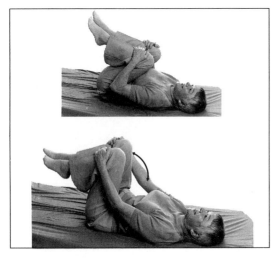

4. Inhale, letting the knees come out away from the chest.
5. Enjoy this movement for two minutes.
6. Breathe into the lower abdomen, moving the energy out the rectum. Feel the lower back relax and the rectum open with each breath.

Benefits: This exercise helps to relieve lower back pains, aches or stiffness, sciatica, constipation, urinary disorders, poor digestion, overeating, belching, snoring, groaning, and fatigue. The following chart lists the acupressure points that are stimulated in the "Knees to the Chest" exercise and each of their traditional benefits.

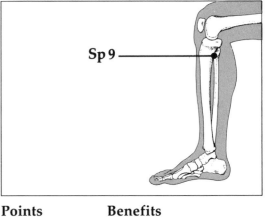

Points	Benefits
Spleen 9	Arthritic knee pains, heavy abdomen, edema.
Stomach 36	Indigestion, abdominal pain, or swelling.

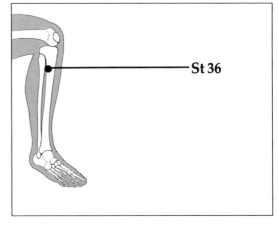

Points	Benefits
Bladder 45	Middle back pain and spasms, abdominal distension.
Bladder 21, 22	Lower backache, stomachache, indigestion, abdominal pain.
Bladder 25	Arthritis in the lower back, constipation, intestinal gas.

Lower Back Twist

1. Begin on your back with your legs bent, feet flat on the floor.
2. Exhale as your knees fall to the left and turn your head to the right.

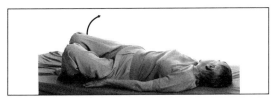

3. Inhale as you bring both your knees up to the center.
4. Exhale and let your knees roll to the right and turn your head to the left.
5. Continue several more times, alternating sides and breathing with the movement.

Benefits: This movement gently stretches the lower back. It also helps to readjust the lower spine.

Caution: This exercise is not recommended for severe lower back problems, such as a ruptured disc. Please consult your osteopath, chiropractor, or physical therapist if you have any questions.

Rock and Roll

Do this exercise while lying on a padded surface.

1. Bring your arms underneath your thighs and clasp one wrist.
2. Bring your knees to your chest and lean back, tucking your head into the chest.

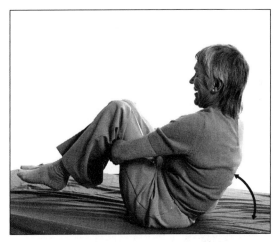

3. Rock back and forth from the base of the spine to the tops of the shoulders. Use the weight of your legs to propel the body back and forth. Inhale coming up, exhale as you go back.

Benefits: Rocking on the spine in this way works on all 94 traditional acupressure points on the back. Try rocking back and forth for one full minute to relieve back pain, tension, and fatigue. Immediately after doing this exercise, relax on your back with your eyes closed for a couple of minutes to enhance the benefits.

RELIEVING SEVERE LOWER BACK PAIN

If you have severe lower back pain, follow the instructions for the Acu-Yoga exercises Flattening the Lower Back and Warming the Vitals. Gradually work toward practicing the other exercises in this section, which are helpful for lower backaches, stiffness, and tension. Remember to breathe deeply, as instructed.

Legs on a Chair

1. Lie on your back, resting your lower legs on a chair with your knees bent. For maximum relief, you should relax in this position for ten to fifteen minutes, breathing slowly and deeply without moving your spine.

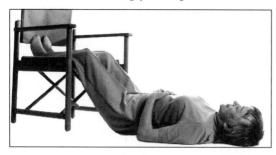

2. Afterwards, lie on your side and bend your knees to your chest until you have completely relaxed for five minutes. Hot pads and compresses are also helpful for relaxing muscular spasms and for improving circulation.

Suggestion: Alternating between cold packs and hot compresses is also helpful for relaxing muscular spasms and for improving circulation. See your chiropractor or doctor for individual medical advice.

Flattening the Lower Back

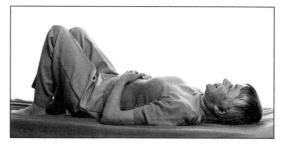

1. Lie on your back with your legs bent and your feet on the floor.
2. Inhale, then exhale, contracting your buttock muscles and pulling in your abdomen so that your lower back presses against the floor. Repeat this several times.

Benefits: This exercise flattens and elongates the lower back to help relieve arthritis in this area. It is excellent for preventing lower backaches if there are no problems with protruding vertebrae or degenerating lumbar discs.

Warming the Vitals

1. Lie on your back with your knees bent and feet flat on the floor. Place your hands one on top of the other, under the sacrum at the base of the spine. Breathe deeply into your lower abdomen for one minute.

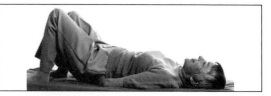

2. Deeply relax with your hands by your sides and your eyes closed to discover the benefits.

ABDOMINAL STRENGTHENING EXERCISES

It is important to strengthen your abdominal muscles in order to stabilize your spinal column. Once a person with a "bum back" begins to tone and strengthen the abdominal muscles, he or she will often feel a general relief of lower back pain and pressure. Try to regularly practice a couple of the following exercises, slowly building up the amount of time you spend on each one.

Swimming

Swimming is excellent for naturally strengthening your abdominal muscles and flattening your belly. The sidestroke and the freestyle stroke are excellent aerobic exercises for strengthening your lower back. Using a kick board is not advisable for people with lower back weakness because it tends to over-accentuate the curve in the lower back.

Pretend Swimming
(with a very slow kick)

1. Lie down on a firm bed, mat, or clean carpeted floor, with a pillow underneath your stomach.
2. Your hands can be by your sides or bent comfortably near your face; your feet ought to remain together.
3. Place either your chin or your forehead on the surface you are lying on.
4. Inhale and raise one leg up. Exhale as you slowly lower it down.
5. Once again, inhale and raise your other leg upward.
6. Continue alternating legs, inhaling up and exhaling down for a minute or two. Then completely relax with your eyes closed as you breathe deeply into your belly to discover the benefits.

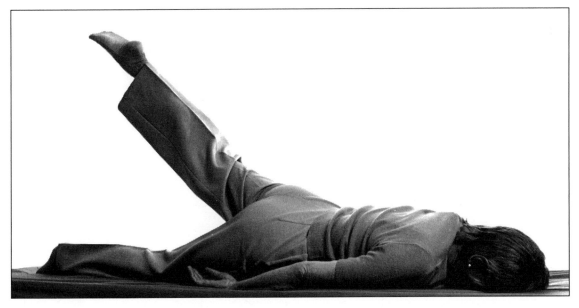

Special Sit-ups for the Lower Back

The following is a progression of abdominal strengthening exercises. Each one should be practiced daily for a week. Begin with the easiest variation for the first week and progress each week to the more difficult exercises.

Caution: While performing these exercises, do not try to rise quickly to a sitting position with a fast, abrupt movement.

Week I

1. Sit up with your knees bent, your feet close together and flat on the floor.

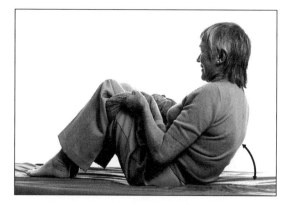

2. Place a towel behind your knees and hold onto the ends of the towel. If a towel is not available, then hold onto your knees.
3. Slowly roll backward until you are at a 45-degree angle from the floor and inhale deeply. Hold for a couple of seconds.
4. Then exhale and sit up again. Repeat this exercise several times until you feel tired.

Week II

Practice the same exercise as Week I except without holding on with your hands. Let your arms simply relax by your sides as you inhale backward to a 45-degree angle and exhale to an upright position.

Week III

Practice the sit-ups with your hands interlaced behind your head. Continue the exercise in this way until you feel tired.

Bridge Pose

1. Lie on your back.
2. Bend your knees so that the soles of your feet are flat on the floor.
3. Put your arms above your head on the floor and relax them.

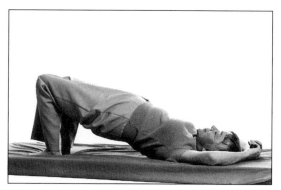

4. Inhale, arching the pelvis up. Hold for several seconds.
5. Exhale as you slowly come down. Continue to inhale up and exhale down for one minute.
6. Relax on your back with your eyes closed for a few minutes.

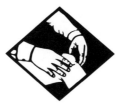

KNEE, HIP, AND SCIATIC PAIN

Arthritis in the hip or knee is often particularly painful since these joints support the weight of the upper body. If you stand on one foot, your body weight — minus the weight of the standing leg — would be resting on your hip and knee joints. When you walk or run, the hip and knee actually have to absorb forces several times the weight of the body — that is, several hundred pounds. Thus when you add arthritis to the great deal of stress and wear on these joints, frequently other surrounding muscle groups may be strained or contracted, resulting in sciatica or back pain and discomfort.

Sciatica refers to a pain that runs down the back of the leg, beginning in the hip or buttock region and traveling down the back of the thigh or along the side of the leg. This pain may extend below the knee and reach as far as the ankle or foot. Pain from sciatica can be intense enough to immobilize someone. Walking or bending in certain directions can be painful. Some people experience numbness in certain areas or pain in the lower back. Sciatic pain can be caused or aggravated by arthritis or a lack of mobility in the pelvic region; lower back strain; excess frustration; injury to the lower back, causing a lumbar disc to protrude; or a misalignment of the sacroiliac joint or lower lumbar region.

Certain exercises help to maintain muscles' length, making them more efficient and stronger than muscles that have been allowed to shorten. Brisk walking, while freely swinging your arms by your sides, is one of the best exercises for lengthening and strengthening the muscles of weight-bearing joints. Arthritics tend to walk slowly; but slow walking, even if done for longer periods of time than brisk walking, does not effectively exercise the muscles through their full range, nor is maximum force exerted on the muscles. Since the weakened muscles of an arthritic patient can lead to decreased activity and mobility, the self-care exercises in this section can be extremely helpful for the leg and pelvic areas.

CAUSES OF BACK, HIP, AND SCIATIC PAIN

Muscular tension and spasms in the lower back and pelvis can be a direct source of sciatica, hip, and lower back pain. Approximately 36 muscles attach to the pelvis, acting together to stabilize the pelvic girdle in relation to the spine. When these muscles are tense or become chronically rigid, spinal nerves in the lower lumbar region can become pinched, blocking circulation and eventually contributing to spinal disc problems and sciatic pain. The following are some of the conditions that can contribute to tension in the pelvis and cause hip pain. *Restrictive Clothing:* Fashion strongly influences how we carry ourselves, which unfortunately is usually in an unhealthy way. For example, it is fashionable to appear slim. As people tighten or hold in their stomachs in an attempt to meet the fashion "ideal," a great deal of pelvic and abdominal tension can result. Tight pants and other tapered clothes which are cut to highlight this slim look, add to the problem. The result is tension, decreased flexibility and mobility in the pelvis, and impaired functioning of the pelvic organs.

Poor Posture and Lack of Movement:
The pelvis is designed to move in all directions. A sedentary lifestyle, in which sitting at desks, riding in cars, and waiting in lines are all common routines, stagnates the body since it does not have an opportunity to be fully moved and stretched. This lack of movement becomes a permanent pattern, tension builds, and the body becomes more and more tight and congested. Posture suffers as a result, since the entire skeletal frame is being thrown out of alignment.

You can see how common this problem is by simply noticing how few people have fluid, strong posture, and how many have their knees locked, pelvises protruding backward (producing a sway-back) and shoulders hunched up. Under the brunt of this bad posture, the pelvis becomes rigid, almost locked into one position. This impairs circulation, weakens genital functioning, and can cause constipation, lumbago, and sciatica.

Chest and Shoulder Tension: There is a direct relationship between tension in the upper and lower portions of the spine. When one portion is out of proper alignment, a strain is put on the other to compensate, so that you end up with tension and poor alignment in both areas. Since most people are more aware of their shoulder tension than their pelvic tension, it is important to work on the pelvis to cultivate an awareness of the tension

stored there.

The depth of the breath is also a barometer for pelvic arthritis and tension. Breathing cannot be full and deep if there is tension in the chest or abdominal and pelvic areas.

Emotional Associations: The pelvis is also considered the gate of the abdomen, where we experience our "gut level" feelings. Abdominal tensions can block off these feelings so that we tend to lose touch with our true needs and desires. Our emotions and their expressions are inhibited by tension and repression. This, of course, results in frustration, since no matter what we do, our deep needs remain unmet.

Many people are stuck in this frustration. The substitute "gratifications" they turn to in an attempt to relieve this frustration are usually destructive habits, such as smoking, drinking, overeating, or eating nonnutritional foods solely for taste or sensation. These habits not only do not satisfy the person, but they also weaken and toxify the body, making the true satisfaction of health and well-being more and more elusive.

Ideally, pelvic tensions, and their associated emotions, are gradually released in a balanced way. Releasing pelvic tension can enable a person to become liberated from anxiety, worry, and fear, and then to more fully experience inner gratification and move forward in life.

RELIEVING HIP/LEG ARTHRITIS AND SCIATICA

Acupressure, along with gentle exercise, is effective for relieving as well as preventing both arthritis in the hip joint and sciatica. Pelvic movements that gently stretch the lower back and buttock muscles complement the highly beneficial therapeutics of acupressure for relieving sciatic pain.

One of my clients who had trouble with hip pain related to the sciatic nerve received tremendous relief from acupressure. Her pain was so acute that she could not lie down flat; she had to prop herself up at night with pillows. I concentrated on pressing the points in the buttocks and lower back, as well as stretching the leg gently to increase flexibility. A series of four acupressure sessions in a ten-day period released the raw, grueling pain she'd had for months. Unfortunately, this client didn't exercise or practice the self-care techniques to follow through on the success of the acupressure sessions, and consequently suffered a recurrence of her hip pain several weeks later. Although she does not work on herself to be pain-free, she now has the security of knowing that professional acupressure sessions can thoroughly relieve her hip pain.

The following Acu-Yoga exercises help to prevent sciatica. They should be practiced twice daily for best results. If you have sciatic pain or a disc problem in your lower back, skip the next exercise. The Hip Rotations can aggravate your existing pain, although they are beneficial for preventing sciatica and lower back-

aches. If you have sciatica, practice the following exercises slowly, with your eyes closed, to increase your awareness. Don't push yourself beyond your limits. Be sure to utilize long, deep breathing.

EXERCISES

Hip Rotations

1. Stand with your feet comfortably spread, about shoulder-width apart.

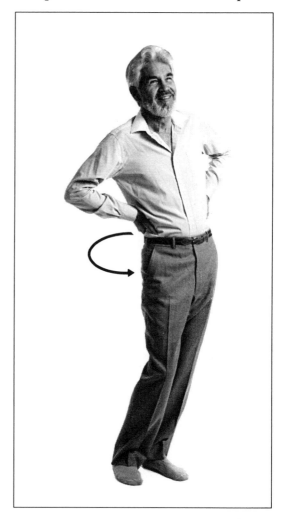

2. Support your lower back on both sides, using your fingertips.
3. Move your hips around in a full circle with your knees slightly bent. Rotate your pelvis several times in one direction, and then in the other. Breathe deeply and enjoy the movement.

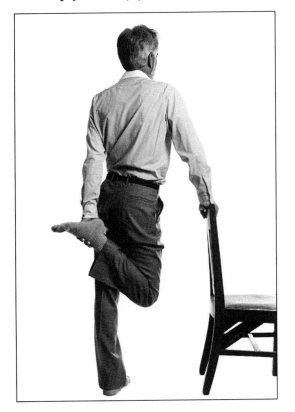

Quad Stretch

1. Hold the back of a chair for support as you stand on your left leg.
2. Bend your right leg and grasp it at the ankle with your left hand. Firmly pull your foot toward your buttocks and hold the stretch for about five to ten seconds. Repeat this stretch on the other leg.

Leg Swing

1. Stand next to a chair, and place your left hand on the back of the chair.

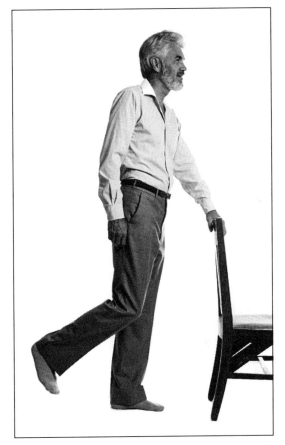

2. Shift all of your weight onto your left foot and swing your right leg freely backward and forward like a pendulum. Make sure you do not swing your leg to the side as this will strain your back.
3. After about thirty seconds, switch sides and swing the other leg. The purpose of this exercise is to promote greater circulation and mobility in the hip joint.

Leg Lifts
For Strengthening the Lower Back[32]

The following Acu-Yoga exercise works on the acupressure points in the pelvic area and can increase the blood supply through the groin, as well as relieve arthritic pain in the hip joint. It is an excellent example of how traditional Yogic postures utilize acupressure, since pressure is directly applied to specific acupressure points in the groin area.

1. Place one large, thick pillow or two flat pillows underneath your abdominal area as you lie down on your stomach. These pillows help prevent the lower back from arching too much.
2. Make fists with your hands and place them under your groin area, with your chin or forehead resting on the floor.
3. Inhale as you raise one leg, and exhale as you lower the leg.

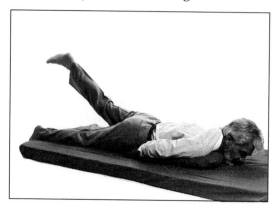

4. Inhale, raising your other leg, and exhale as you lower it.
5. Continue alternating legs for a minute.
6. Then let yourself relax by closing your eyes and taking several long, deep breaths.

Benefits: Relieves arthritis in the hip joint; improves posture, elimination, and digestion; strengthens the immune system, the spleen, and the pancreas. Relieves indigestion, gas, rheumatism, poor leg circulation, and cold feet.

Windshield Wipers
For Leg and Knee Arthritis

1. Lying comfortably on your back with your feet shoulder-width apart, roll your legs inward and outward by bringing your large toes together and then apart.

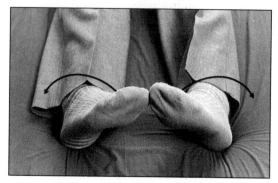

2. Continue rolling your legs for a minute to increase the circulation in the legs and feet.

Important: After practicing these techniques, allow yourself five to ten minutes of deep relaxation, lying on your back with your eyes closed. Remember, relaxation enhances the benefits.

SELF-ACUPRESSURE
For Arthritis in the Hips and Lower Back

1. Roll onto your side. Place your fist or a tennis ball underneath the side of your buttock. This will press the key

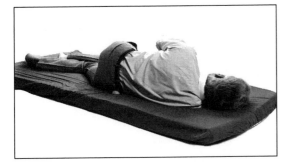

   acupressure point (GB 30) in the center of the buttock for relieving sciatica. The pressure on this point should create a pain that "hurts good." Close your eyes and breathe deeply for several minutes.

2. Lie on your back. Place both fists under your lower back. Position your knuckles underneath your tightest lower back muscles. Breathe deeply with your eyes closed in this position for one minute. Readjust the pressure as the soreness decreases, pressing other tight points in the area.

3. Roll onto your other side and repeat Step 1.

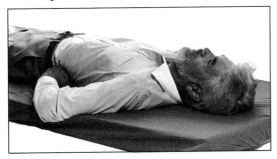

ARTHRITIS RELIEF POINTS[33]

GB 34 is a muscle relaxant point located on the outside of the lower leg, below and in front of the head of the fibula. **GB 40** is in the indentation directly in front of the outer ankle bone.

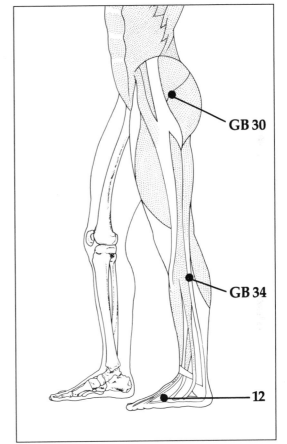

GB 30

GB 34

12

Point #12 is between the fourth and fifth metatarsals below the juncture where the bones begin to narrow on top of the foot.

---

[33] These numbers refer to the acupuncture/acupressure point system of the body. You do not need to know any of these reference numbers to practice the Arthritis Relief Program.

KNEE ARTHRITIS RELIEF
An Isometric Exercise

1. Sitting in a chair, extend one leg straight out so that your foot comes up to the level of your hips.

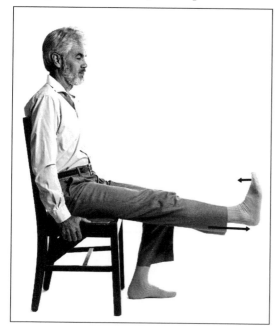

2. Take a couple of long, deep breaths as you flex the toe toward you and your heel pushes away from you. This will tighten and eventually strengthen the quadriceps and can relieve knee pain.
3. Now switch to exercise your opposite leg. Your thigh muscle should feel hard when you lift your leg up to the level of your hips.

Further Suggestions: This is an excellent exercise to practice many times throughout the day. Try it also in bed, both in the morning before rising and at night before going to sleep. Simply extend your legs outward as you lie on your back, and breathe deeply as you flex your toes toward you and stretch your heel away from you.

Points for Relieving Knee Pain

First apply hot compresses with a thick, heavy towel until the heat penetrates deep into the knee joint. For the next few weeks, spend ten minutes three times a day thoroughly massaging the painful knee using the following methods and points. Try to stay off your legs during this time (e.g., avoid stairs as much as possible) to give your knee the necessary rest to enable the joint to heal.

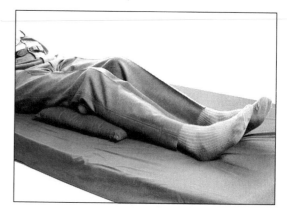

1. Sit on a mat, on a carpet, or in bed with your back supported and your legs extended in front of you. Place a tennis ball in the center of the crease behind your knee. This presses Point B 54, a good point for relieving sciatica, knee, and back pain. If you place a pillow underneath the tennis ball, it will both stabilize the ball from rolling and comfortably support your bent knee.

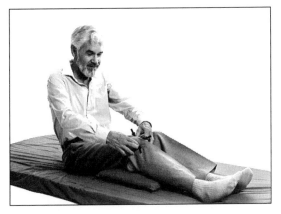

2. Firmly press or briskly rub the following points while the tennis ball is positioned in the center of the crease behind your knee.[34]

Lv 8 is in the inside of the knee joint. Feel for the groove formed when the knee is bent.
B 53 is on the outside of the crease behind the knee.

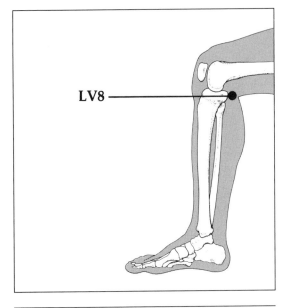

LV8

---

[34] Do not rub your leg if you have a blood clot.

K 1 is in the center of the bottom of the foot.
St 35 is in the indentation between the kneecap and the shinbone when the knee is bent.

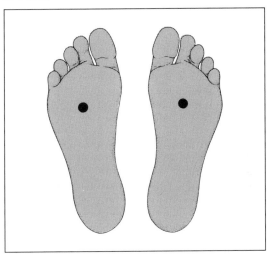

St 36 is on the outer side of the calf, four finger-widths below the knee, a half-inch out from the shinbone.

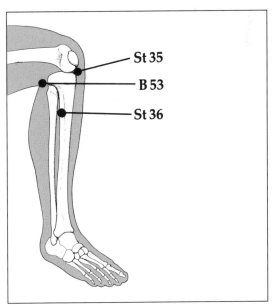

St 35
B 53
St 36

Edema Points

Edema is a local or generalized condition in which the body tissues contain an excessive amount of fluid. It is caused by increased permeability of capillary walls and/or by increased capillary pressure. The following two acupressure points are especially beneficial for balancing the swelling and for pain in the knees or legs.

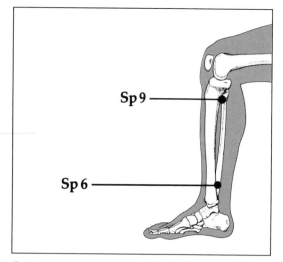

Sp 6 is approximately four finger-widths above the inside ankle bone, on the back border of the shinbone.

Sp9 is on the inside of the leg below the knee (under the medial condyle of the tibia). Press into an indentation in the bone, angling your pressure upward.

Patient Care: Hold Sp 6 and Sp 9.

Benefits: "Water on the knee," swollen ankles, abdominal distention, poor circulation, cold feet, diabetes, extreme fatigue, general weakness, irregular menstruation, knee problems.

TECHNIQUES FOR HELPING OTHERS WITH LOWER BACK, HIP, KNEE, AND SCIATIC PAIN

A medical doctor should first be seen for a complete physical examination and diagnosis, since spinal problems, cancer, and diabetes can have many of the same symptoms. However, if your sciatic pain is the result of a minor misalignment, muscular spasm, or a deformation of the spine due to aging, then receiving a few of the following acupressure sessions, accompanied by a nap or deep relaxation immediately afterward, can bring relief.

With recipient lying on his or her stomach:

1. Apply hot compresses (preferably using ginger water)[35] to the lower back and sacrum. Use two thick towels and alternate them to keep the compresses constantly hot (at a bearable temperature).

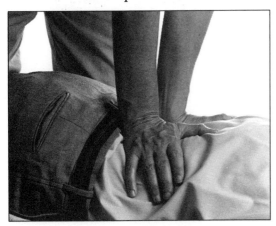

2. Using the palms of your hands on the lower back and buttocks, lean your weight on Points #10 and B 48 to apply pressure for one minute each.

3. Use your thumbs to gradually apply about five seconds of firm pressure on each of the points in the lower back and sacral areas, as illustrated.[36]

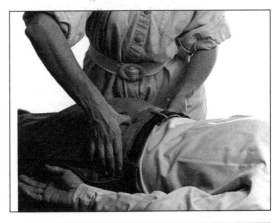

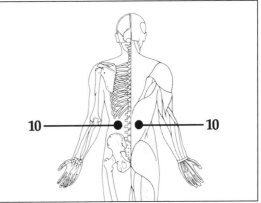

---

[35] See page 201 in the "Self-Help Tools" chapter for specific instructions on how to prepare ginger compresses.

[36] If the recipient is very sensitive to acupressure or if the sciatica is chronic, then try to stimulate the same points with heat from a hand-held dryer.

4. Again use the palms of your hands and lean your weight into the center of the back of the leg.[37] Start at the crease where the buttocks meet the top of the thighs and progress down inch by inch to the ankles.

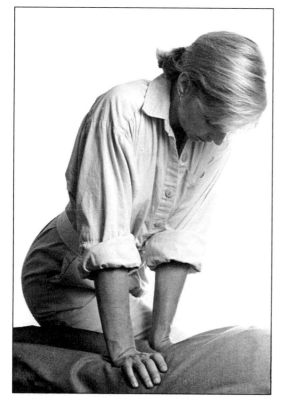

5. Go over the same area behind the leg, but this time use your thumbs, especially on the specific points illustrated.

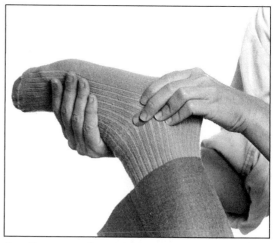

6. Squeeze the ankles and press GB 40 in the hollow space directly in front of the outer ankle bone.

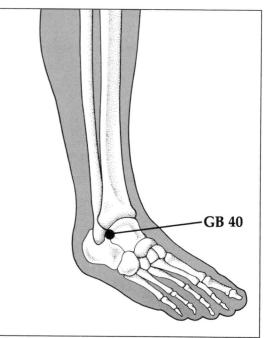

---

[37] Be careful not to press the kneecap into the floor when you press the back of the knee.

With recipient lying on his or her back:

7. Kneel close to the outside of the recipient's right thigh. Use your left hand to pick up the leg from underneath the knee as you support the recipient's foot with your right hand.

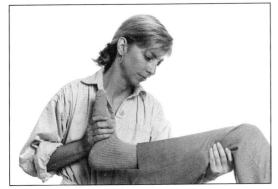

8. Gradually bring the knee toward the chin. Instruct the recipient to breathe long and deep as you rotate the knee in a slow, circular motion, first in one direction and then the other. Begin with small movements, then gradually increase the size of the circle.

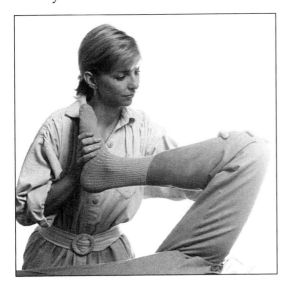

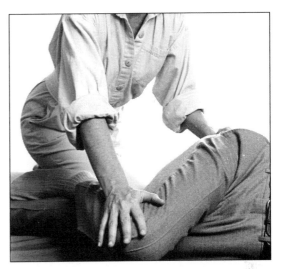

9. Finish the movement by slowly bringing the right knee over to the left side of the recipient to twist and stretch the lower back. Do not make any fast or jarring movements.

10. Slowly stretch the muscles in the hips and lower back, then lower the right leg to the ground. Repeat the rotation on the left side, allowing three to five minutes per side.

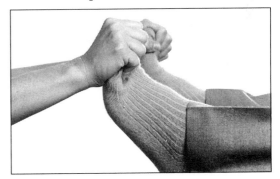

11. End the session by grasping the toes of both feet. Hold firmly for one or two minutes to end with a simple acupressure method that balances both sides of the body.

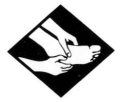

FOOT AND
ANKLE PAIN

It is extremely important to maintain flexibility in the feet and ankles. We depend on their flexing to compensate for the unevenness of the ground and to carry the weight of our bodies as we alternate from one foot to the other. With pain and stiffness in the feet and ankles, standing and moving are difficult, and the body is often thrown out of balance. Another result is undue stress placed on the hips and knees, which can lead to degenerative osteoarthritis.

The foot, ankle, knee, and hip all combine to absorb the impact of force when we walk or jump. The two flexible arches of the foot — traverse (metatarsal arch) and the longitudinal arch — together with the muscles of the ankle, respond to each step we take.

Anatomically, the feet are similar to the hands. Instead of the *carpal* bones of the hand, we have the much larger *tarsal*

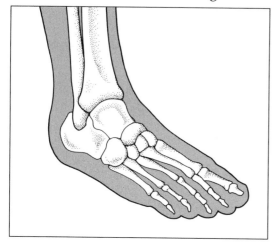

bones of the feet. There are five *metatarsal* bones which are joined to the phalanges of the five toes, forming the metatarsal phalangeal (MTP) joints.

In rheumatoid arthritis, the MTP joints are subject to attack, and deformities in the feet result that are similar to those in the MTP joints of the hands. The big toe turns in toward the other toes and no longer contributes adequate strength to the push-off part of a walking step. There are various supports and splints available to remedy the situation; however, exercise and massage can delay the need for more radical measures, while increasing flexibility of the foot.

One of my older clients, who had arthritis in her foot and ankle as well as in her hands, told me that her acupressure sessions were worth "a million dollars." Because she lived a long distance away, she could only see me occasionally. Her ankle had swelled up and she had pain on the top of her foot that extended down into many of her toes. According to her, the acupressure sessions not only relieved her pain, but also kept her feeling better for over three weeks at a time.

Another client of mine had a consistent dull, aching pain on the top of her foot. The arthritic pain and stiffness made it difficult for her to walk. I used the acupressure points located between the bones on the top of the feet, with a slow, firm massage. Then I gently stretched the foot to increase her circulation and flexibility. Pressure on the reflexology points on the bottom of the feet (see the chart in this chapter) also gave her tremendous relief.

The following routine is a combination of exercise and massage to help keep the foot flexible and strong. Exercising and massaging the muscles around the ankle will help ensure that you maintain a good range of motion and will also help prevent future joint problems.

The Chinese long ago recognized the importance of the feet to the total health of the body. I do share the belief that the health of the entire skeletal system benefits when the feet are kept supple. I have noticed that if I experience pain in my feet while walking — let us say due to a painful metatarsal arch — I tend to pull my shoulders up and my neck becomes stiff.[38]

STRENGTHENING THE TOES

1. Try offering resistance to the tip of each toe, pressing it against a finger or some other object.

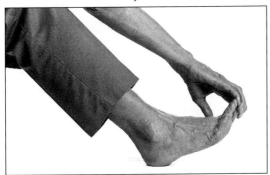

2. Practice curling your toes by picking up a pencil with your toes or grasping a piece of cloth with your toes and pulling against the resistance.
3. Use your hands to spread and extend your toes upward as far as possible for a good range-of-motion exercise.

[38] Semyon Krewer, *The Arthritis Exercise Book,* Simon & Schuster, 1981.

HYDROTHERAPY FOR THE FEET

Hot foot baths once or twice a day are highly recommended for people with rheumatoid arthritis. The heat increases the circulation and helps to relief stiffness. Try a foot bath just before doing your daily exercises, before having company, or just before going out for a walk, running some errands, or going out for dinner. Simply let your feet soak for ten to fifteen minutes. Occasionally you might try using a commercial foot-bath powder, mineral salts, or bath oil for an extra treat.

Caution: A hot foot bath may cause dizziness upon standing. Therefore, rise slowly to maintain your balance.

Swollen Feet

Arthritics often have an excess of fluids in their feet. Walking or standing on your feet for long periods of time tends to cause the feet to swell. Lying down for long periods of time — e.g., at night — can cause sluggishness in the lymphatic fluids. Next time you get swollen feet, try the following vibrating exercises and self-acupressure points on the ankles.

Sitting in a comfortable chair:

1. Rotate your feet at the ankle joints several times in one direction; then rotate in the opposite direction.

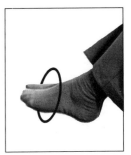

2. Lift one foot off the ground and briskly shake it from side to side for ten to fifteen seconds. Repeat this with your other foot.

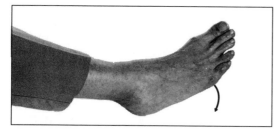

3. Lift one foot up again, then rapidly shake it up and down as you count to ten and then take a deep breath. Repeat this with your other foot.

4. Now place both feet underneath your seat, bending your knees and keeping your toes on the ground. Rapidly shake your heels, bringing them together and apart for twenty to thirty seconds.

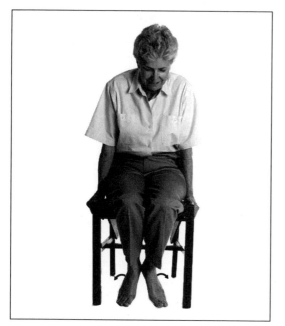

5. Place one of your feet on your opposite knee to hold the points K 6 (on the inside of the ankle) and B 62 (on the outer ankle) as shown.

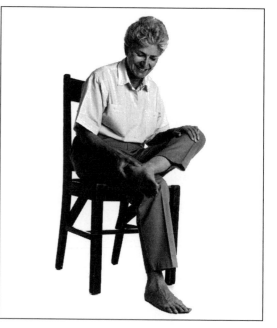

a. Hold these points for a minute and then switch positions so that you can hold the points on your other ankle.

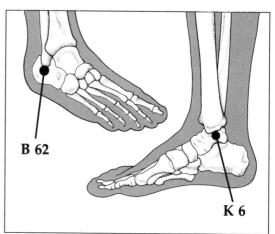

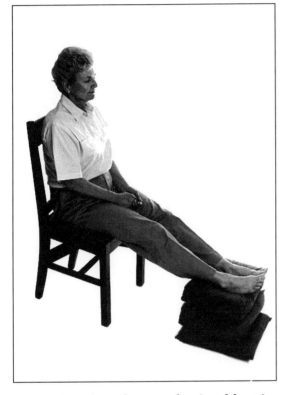

b. Finish with several enjoyable minutes of relaxation. Put your feet up on a chair, close your eyes, and breathe deeply as you let your entire body — from your shoulders to your ankles — relax.

FOOT REFLEXOLOGY FOR RELIEVING ARTHRITIS

Reflexology, a form of therapeutic foot massage, can be very helpful for relieving arthritic pain not only in the feet, but in all parts of the body. It is based on stimulating the nerve endings on the soles of the feet which trigger benefits to the corresponding arthritic areas. Because many of the body's nerves have endings in the feet, there is a reflex action back to a particular body part (where the nerve originated) when the specific associated area on the foot is stimulated.

The points used in reflexology, which can be applied both to oneself and to others, are similar to the acupressure points except that they follow the neurological instead of bio-electrical pathways. Foot reflexology is especially beneficial for relieving arthritic aches and pains when used in conjunction with acupressure. Several important acupressure points on the feet coincide with the nerve reflex points used in reflexology. The extra pain relief effectiveness is the result of utilizing both of these drug-free, hands-on systems.

The amount of pressure needed in reflexology will vary from person to person and from point to point. The pressure should feel good but should be firm enough to stimulate the point. If the amount of pressure is too much for the person to take, ease up and hold the point more lightly until it releases a bit, and then go a little deeper. For very sore, arthritic spots, gradual prolonged light pressure is best: Touch rather than press these spots. As the point is held, the tension will release and more pressure will be appropriate. In any case, work smoothly and carefully so as not to produce any jarring pain.

People who eat a lot of processed foods and who do not get enough exercise may have many tender spots on their feet. This indicates that the glands, organs, and nerves are in poor condition and that there are blockages in the body. Be sensitive to how the points feel on the person and adjust the pressure accordingly.

Foot massage is especially good for arthritis patients as well as for the elderly, sick, or disabled. It simply feels good, and relaxes and rejuvenates the entire body. It improves the circulation so that toxic materials held in the body can be released, benefiting the blood, organs, glands, and nerves.

Your first reflexology treatments should be a maximum of twenty minutes long. This can be repeated as often as every other day for the first week. Gradually work longer on the points or areas that need special attention, namely the most tender spots. As you gain experience, you will learn how to adjust the pressure and begin to relate these points to specific body parts by referring to the reflexology charts.

An excellent natural way to massage the reflexology points on the feet is to walk barefoot as much as possible. Walking on grass, sand, earth, or smooth rocks naturally stimulates these points and also enables the body to absorb the subtle electrical energies of the earth. If the soles of your feet are especially tender, it's best to walk barefoot on grass or soft earth, gradually increasing the time until your feet are stronger.

The reflexology points lie underneath the skin. Note that the size of the points varies, with some covering an area the size of a kidney bean and others no bigger than the head of a pin. Develop your sensitivity to the points through attentive practice.

FOOT REFLEXOLOGY CHART

When there is joint inflammation or an imbalance in an area of the body, it will register in the corresponding areas of the feet. Crystallized calcium deposits tend to accumulate over the nerve endings where these reflex points are located.[39] Press on these points to break up and dissolve the deposits. Pressure on these reflexology points also stimulates the corresponding nerves to relieve pain and balance the affected area of the body.

[39] Kevin and Barbara Kunz, *The Complete Guide for Foot Reflexology*, Prentice Hall Press, 1982.
Note: The Kunz's books are all excellent. For more information write: Reflexology Research Project, Box 35820, Stn. D., Albuquerque, NM 87176.

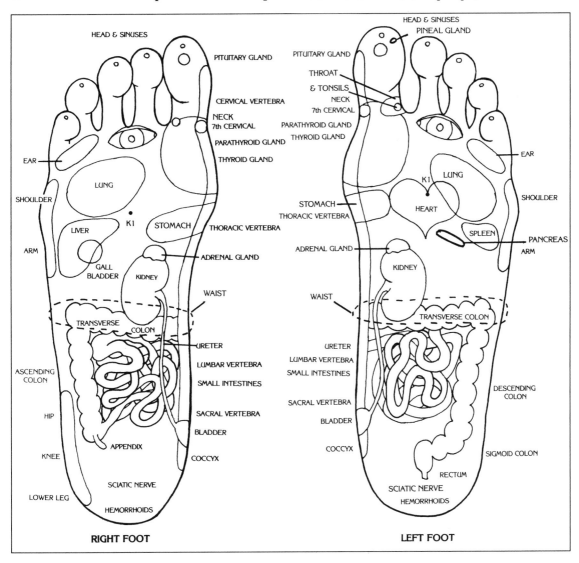

RIGHT FOOT   **LEFT FOOT**

ACUPRESSURE POINT CHART

Instructions for Applying Pressure

When there is an imbalance or a joint inflammation in the body, it will register in a corresponding area on the foot. Use between one and five pounds of pressure on these points. Gradual prolonged pressure is most effective for relieving arthritis in all parts of the body. The massage or pressure applied should feel good, somewhere between pain and pleasure.

The following Foot Acupressure Point Chart illustrates all of the acupressure points on the top and sides of the feet. This reference chart will help you find these key trigger points that help to relieve arthritis. Explore these points as you practice the foot massage instructions and suggestions that follow.

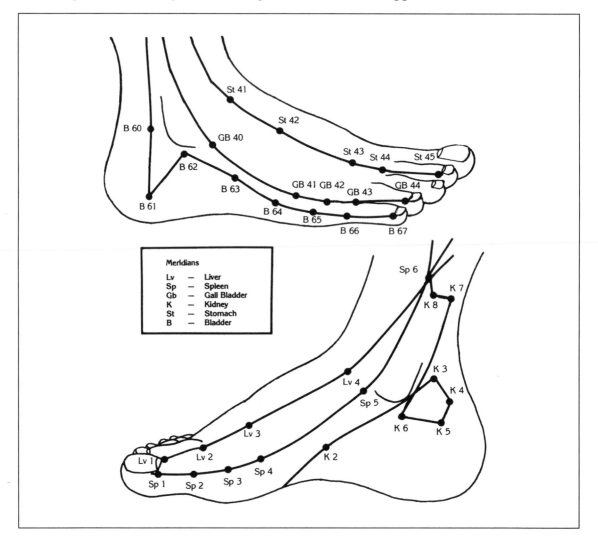

Meridians

Lv	—	Liver
Sp	—	Spleen
Gb	—	Gall Bladder
K	—	Kidney
St	—	Stomach
B	—	Bladder

SELF-MASSAGE TECHNIQUES

Foot Massage Suggestions

- **_Work with an instrument_**, such as an avocado pit or a golf ball, especially if you have arthritis in your hands. Keep your fingernails cut fairly short.

- **_Close your eyes_** in order to more fully relax, and to enjoy and discover the benefits while you give yourself a foot massage.

- **_Avoid distractions_** when possible. Adjust the light so it is not too bright, and make sure you are warm and comfortable.

- **_Ease up_** on the areas that are most sore or painful, and hold them longer to erase the pain and promote healing.

- **_Breathe deeply_** rather than tense up if a point is especially sensitive to touch.

- **_Concentrate_** on what you are doing. Keep your attention focused on your body's signals in the present moment.

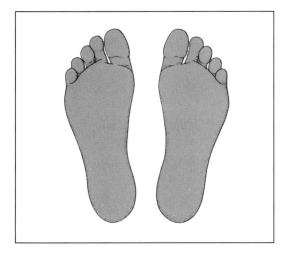

Foot Massage Instructions

The following self-help foot massage can also be practiced on others. Work on one foot at a time.

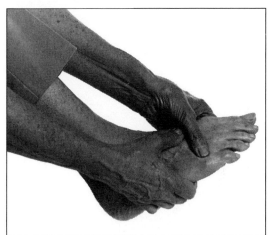

1. Rub and squeeze the foot with your fingers and palms. Massage the entire foot. This is especially good for relieving fatigue as well as generalized aches and pains.

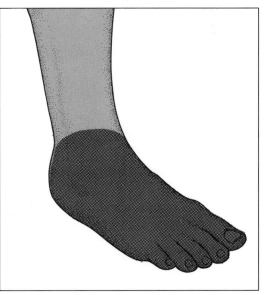

2. Press the points on the arch with your thumb or knuckles, beginning near the heel and working toward the large toe. This stimulates the reflexes of the spine to help relieve arthritis in the back.

3. When you reach the base of the big toe, rub and press that area in a circular direction; it will be about the size of an almond. This affects the stomach and thyroid gland reflexes.

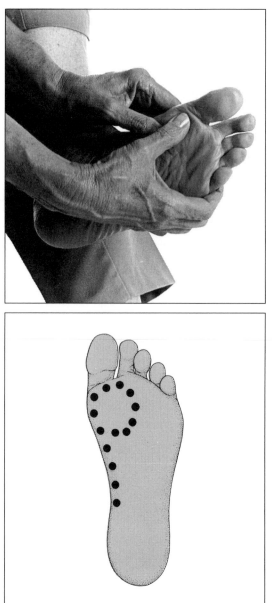

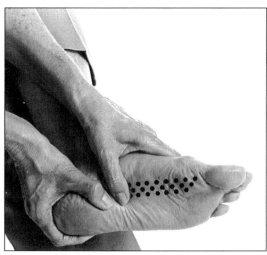

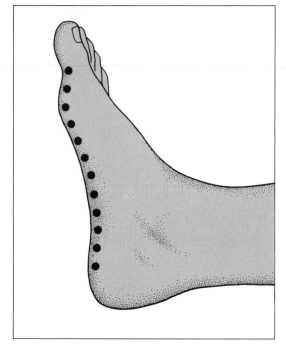

4. Next, massage all of the toes well, pressing the reflex points corresponding to the brain and neck. Using your fingers and thumbs in a pinching position, lightly massage and pinch the skin between the toes. Also, pressing the base of the toes is helpful for arthritis in the neck. It also stimulates the reflexes to the eyes, throat, and back of the head for relieving headaches and congestion.

5. Using both of your thumbs, massage and press the entire sole of the foot. Systematically cover this area where the reflexes to all of the internal organs are located.

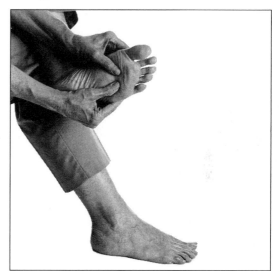

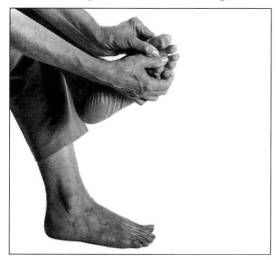

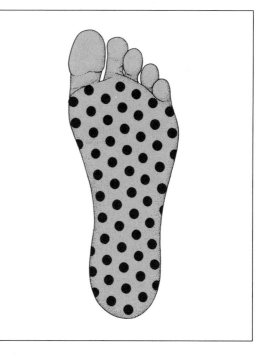

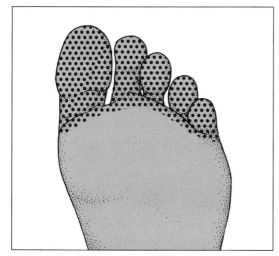

6a. Knead and pinch the outsides of your feet with your thumbs and index fingers. This area represents the joints and therefore is especially good for relieving arthritic aches and pains.

6b. Now press and massage between the bones on the top of the foot. The sore spots you find here correspond to the joints of both the hands and feet.

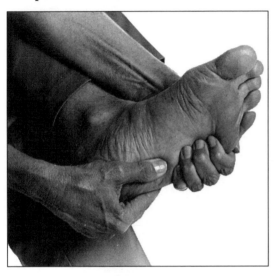

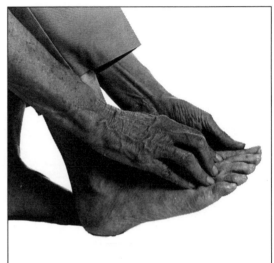

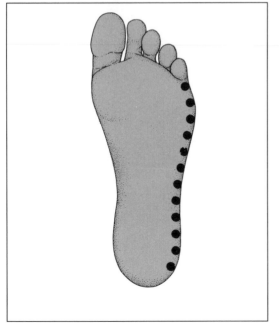

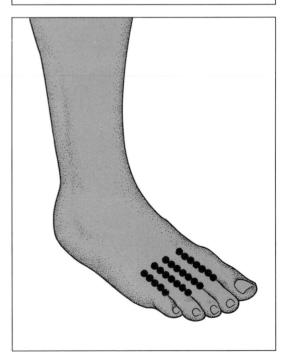

7a. Next, work on the inner and outer heel areas. Pinch and press the grooves and indentations of the heel, ankle, and top of the instep. These areas traditionally have been used to promote relaxation and a good night's sleep. These points also benefit the bladder, kidneys, and reproductive organs.

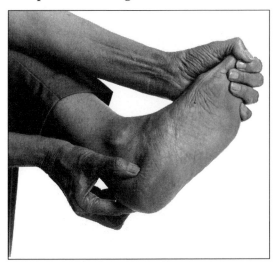

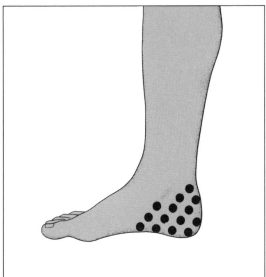

7b. Massage the bottom and sides of the heel, including the ankles. This area relates to the pelvis, sacrum, sciatic nerve, rectum, and sex organs. In traditional Chinese medicine, this area of the foot is used to help relieve hemorrhoids and to promote their healing.

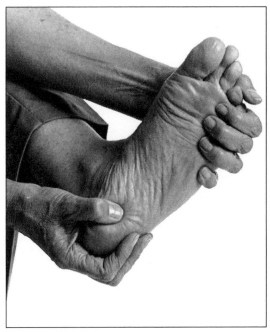

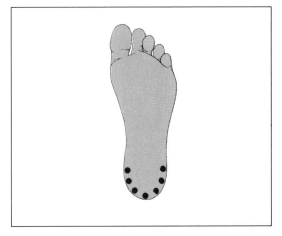

8. Squeeze the Achilles tendon — the cord behind the heel that attaches to the calf muscle. Pinch and knead this tendon from the insertion into the heel all the way up to the base of the calf muscle. This is beneficial for sore or swollen ankles as well as for preventing "charley horses," cramping in the calf muscles.

9. Place your feet flat on the ground, and work on the tops of the feet, massaging in between the bones. Carefully explore the acupressure points on the top of the foot as you press firmly on these digestive aid points located between the bones that attach to the toes.

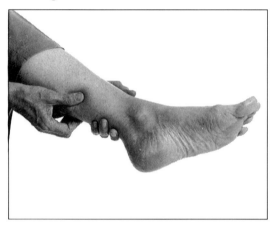

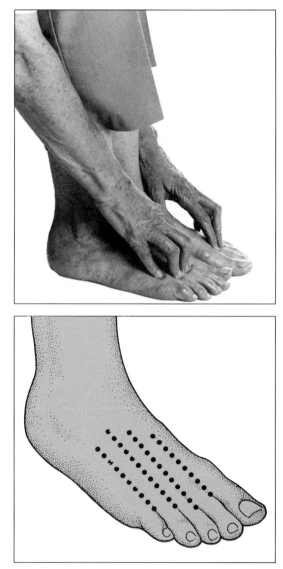

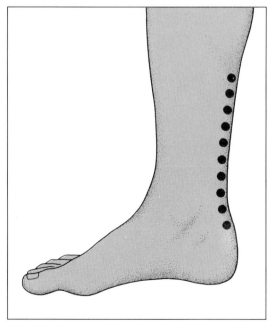

10. With your feet still on the ground, bend each toe upward. Stretch each toe one at a time, bending it at a 90-degree angle from the ground. This stimulates and benefits the circulation.

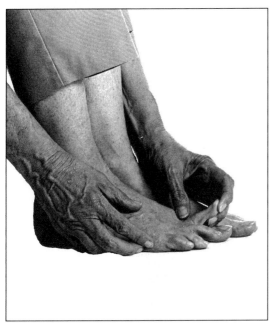

11. Gently spread each toe apart. Be gentle, because the skin between each toe is delicate. Then press and massage the webbing between the toes, which corresponds with the sensory organs in the reflexology system.

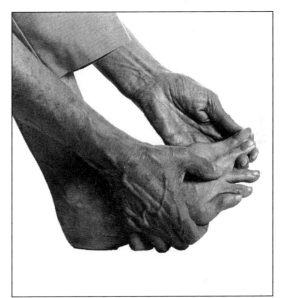

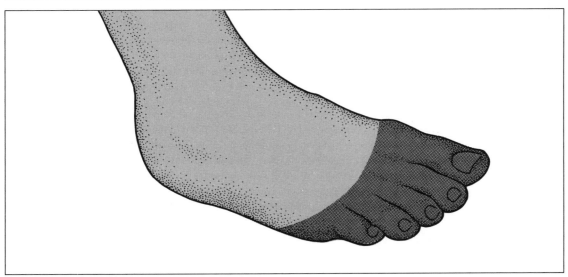

12. Enclose the toes of one foot in the palm of your hand and stretch the toes down. This will often crack the toes properly to release pressure in the joints. Then carefully interlace your fingers in between each of the toes and firmly squeeze a few times. Release this position as you breathe deeply to discover the benefits.

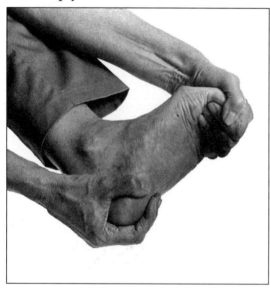

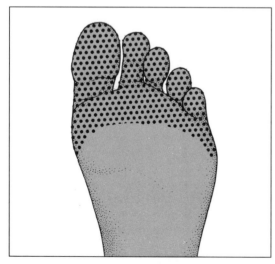

13. Massage the bottoms and arches of the feet with both of your thumbs. Press and pull out each toe. Make the whole foot feel vibrant and alive.

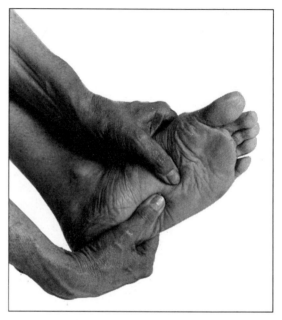

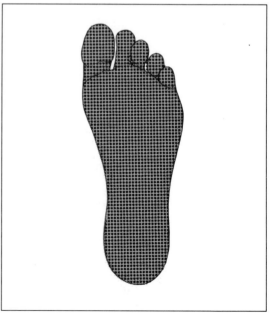

14. Lastly, grasp the whole foot and wring it out like a washrag. Switch hands and wring it out again. Also wring out your ankle a couple of times in both directions. Finish by gently massaging the toes.

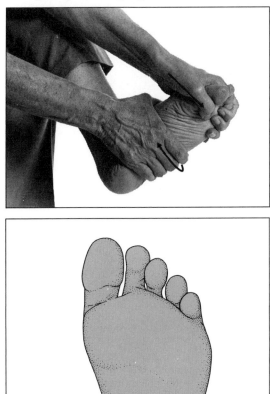

Before you go on and work on the other foot, close your eyes for a minute. Wiggle your toes and compare the different feelings of your two feet. Breathe deeply and enhance the relaxation as you repeat these steps on the other foot. After you give yourself a few minutes to relax with your feet propped up, see if the areas of your arthritis are relieved. From here, you can focus on treating yourself in ways that will *maintain* this sense of well-being that is rightfully yours.

FOOT MASSAGE BALL

While sitting comfortably in a chair, try rolling a golf ball or avocado pit back and forth across the bottom of each foot. If you find a golf ball is too hard, try using the "foot massage ball-roller" while wearing thick socks, or try using a tennis ball. To keep the ball in place, it is best to do the rolling on a carpeted surface. Try using the foot massage ball after taking a hot bath, shower, or foot bath. You will find it an easy, enjoyable way to help yourself at home while watching television, talking on the phone, or reading.

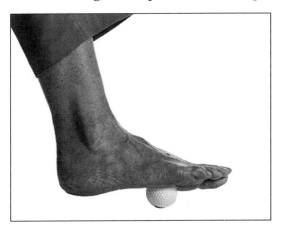

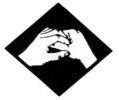

CHAPTER VII

POOR CIRCULATION

POOR CIRCULATION

During arthritic pain, muscular tension blocks proper circulation. The contracted muscular tissue physically constricts the arteries and veins, and therefore constricts the flow of blood. Involuntary, chronic tensions caused by tensing against arthritic pain can block circulation even further.

A majority of circulation problems are caused by muscular tension and a lack of exercise. Exercise stimulates the heart to pump faster and stronger, increasing circulation to get the necessary oxygen to the cells of the body. Physical exercise moves the body, warms it up, stretches and loosens tendons, and releases tension in the muscles.

Poor circulation is a self-perpetuating, negative condition. That is, if an area is imbalanced so that the circulatory flow is impeded, then the lack of circulation itself causes further imbalances. When the blood cannot properly get to the cells to bring oxygen and nutrients and to flush away waste material, then the cells and tissues become undernourished; toxins accumulate, thus furthering the stagnation and tension in the area.

Over four thousand years ago, *The Yellow Emperor's Classic of Internal Medicine* described the circulation of the blood, which was not discovered by Western physicians until the sixteenth century. Since ancient times, acupressure and exercise techniques have been used in the Orient to improve circulation.

Acu-Yoga, the combination of using acupressure and gentle stretching, improves circulation in two ways. First, by applying pressure directly on the acupressure points, where tension collects, the muscles in that area will be able to relax. Second, as a highly developed form of physical exercise, Acu-Yoga stretches the muscles and moves all parts of the body. Through daily practice, the elasticity of the arteries can improve. The combination of acupressure and yoga opens the blood flow so that fresh nutrients can circulate in painful, swollen joints, and toxins and other acidic wastes can be carried off for excretion.

During cold weather, people with poor circulation feel uncomfortably cold, and there is a tendency, unfortunately, to tighten up. Of course it is the exact opposite that brings relief, namely relaxing with the cold. When you tighten against cold, you simply create more tension and thus less circulation. The next time you are cold, take big, deep breaths and let yourself RELAX! Move your body, breathe, and feel the circulation of the blood and energy. Fighting the cold does not work. Flowing with it does!

Circulation problems are commonly

caused by both mental as well as physical stress. Simple mental exercises such as meditation and visualization can be very effective for relaxing the mind. Once the mind is at ease, the body can then easily relax. The release of tension through focusing on positive thoughts and images increases the circulation and relieves pain. A deep relaxation naturally results from practicing the following mental exercises, which often promotes pain relief, stress reduction, and mental clarity.

MEDITATION

The stillness achieved during meditation also slows down the metabolism of the body. This provides a deep state of rest which has great therapeutic benefits; it relaxes the muscles as well as rejuvenates the entire body, especially the nerves and joints.

One important purpose of meditation is to use your mental facilities for sharpening concentration, and at the same time you can expand to higher levels of awareness. This can be accomplished by focusing your mind, which allows you to temporarily step aside from its constant chatter. The mind can then go beyond its normal scope into a vastness that is tremendously beneficial for relieving arthritic pain and for helping your body to rebalance and heal itself.

Most people operate from a surface shell, a mentality that protects them and limits their scope. Over the years, the mind can become rigid and partially dysfunctional, just as the joints can become stiff and inflexible with age.

Meditation is a stress reduction skill that can enable you to balance the sides of your brain, relax your mind, and at the same time sharpen your concentration and memory. Like anything worthwhile, it requires effort and some self-discipline to achieve these marvelous results. Actually, the benefits of this inner mental work are so rewarding that a meditation practice becomes a joy, not a duty or an exercise. With practice, meditation can make your life easier, more fulfilling, and can expand it in ways you never imagined.

Breathing Meditation for Pain Relief
1. Sit comfortably in a firm chair with your spine straight, and close your eyes.

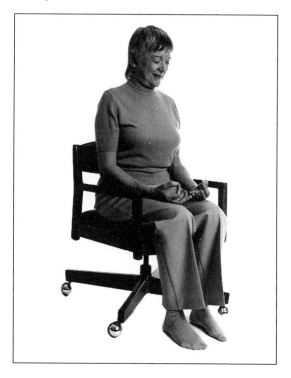

2. Gently lift your chest and press your chin lightly into the hollow of your throat.

3. Connect the tips of the thumb and index finger of each hand, and rest the backs of the hands on your knees.

4. Simply concentrate on breathing deeply into your lower abdomen with your spine straight for at least three minutes. Focus on your breath. Gently control your respiratory system, making each breath grow longer and deeper.

Breathe out any tensions that are restricting your lungs from moving fully and naturally. Feel your mind growing clearer with each breath.

Notice the resistance your mind creates: the barriers of judging and analyzing that it comes up against. Take several deep breaths and let go of the barriers. Breathe deeply and gently, as if you are bringing vital energy into your system.

Hold the breath at the top of the exhalation, feeling its fullness. Exhale smoothly and discover the benefits circulating throughout your body.

If you meditate on the breath in this way as much as possible, it will decrease your aches and pains as well as heighten your memory and increase your effectiveness in life. You can do it any time, even when you are occupied with your daily activities. Put your attention on breathing deeply for a few moments and then experience the benefits it provides.

Mind-Clearing Meditation

1. Sit comfortably in a firm chair with your spine straight.

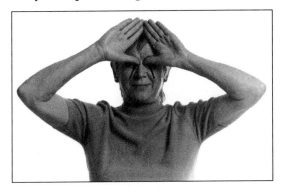

2. Place the pads of your thumbs into the area where the upper ridge of the eye socket joins the bridge of the nose (Bladder 2). Place the fingertips of each hand together.

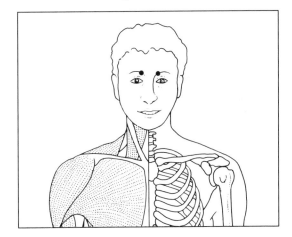

3. Let your elbows point slightly out to the sides, creating an equilateral triangle with your forearms. Close your eyes. Now visualize the pyramid or triangle that you are forming with your arms, and keep your spine straight as you breathe deeply.

4. Sit quietly, letting the power of the meditation increase.

5. After a minute, slowly let your hands relax into your lap. Sit quietly for a couple of minutes with your eyes closed and your spine straight to discover the benefits.

The Mind-Clearing Meditation rebalances the pituitary gland as well as the memory of both painful and pleasant past experiences. An excess of reminiscing about the past can have a damaging effect on your memory. If you get stuck in the past, you may not be alert and able to shift your attention to fully recall information. When you become preoccupied with what happened or what could have happened in the past, you can lose touch with what is presently before you. By exercising your awareness of what is here and now, you gain an attentiveness that can add to your own self-healing.

Dietary Considerations

There are some dietary considerations related to arthritic pain and poor circulation. If your body feels cold, especially your hands or feet, this can be caused by eating too many cold-producing foods. To balance this, limit your intake of alcohol, fruit, honey, soft drinks, frozen food, and fruit juice. Especially be sure to eliminate foods containing white sugar.[40]

Sautéed onion, ginger, and burdock root are three foods that help aid circulation. Miso soup is excellent for improving circulation, general strengthening, and warming up the body.[41] In general, of course, hot foods heat up the body, and cold ones cool it down. However, "spicy hot" foods — chili, curry, etc. — do heat up the body, but they can also be irritants to the system when eaten in excess. Buckwheat is considered one of the most heat-producing vegetarian foods. To achieve balance, as a general rule, all foods should be eaten in moderation.

ACUPRESSURE FOR GREATER CIRCULATION

One of the primary physiological benefits of acupressure is the improvement of circulation. As acupressure releases muscular tension, enabling the blood to flow more freely, the increased circulation benefits arthritic joints, relieves pain, and allows toxins to be released and eliminated. Increased circulation also brings more oxygen and other nutrients to affected muscles and arthritic joints. This helps relieve pain, stimulates healing, and increases resistance to illness, which of course promotes a longer, healthier life.

The following acupressure points are helpful for increasing circulation into specific areas. First, knead or massage the general area where you have poor circulation. Then choose one or more points that are on or near these areas. Do

---

[40] If you have the opposite condition and are generally very warm, intense, and hyperactive, balance this by limiting your intake of meat and salt.

[41] Miso is a traditional Oriental food made from aged soybeans and salt. Consult a health food store for cookbooks with recipes using miso.

this a couple of times a day for two to three minutes (on both sides of your body) using firm pressure. The following instructions will give you the location of the point, how to press it, and the benefits of using the point.

Overall Body Circulation Point: GB 21

Location: On the top edge of the shoulder muscle at the highest point, just one-half inch lateral to where the base of the neck joins the shoulder.

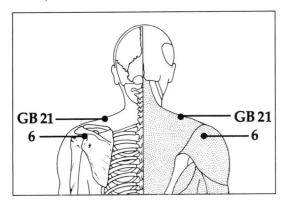

Finger Application: Hold the muscular tension on the top of the shoulder. Gradually ease deeper into the muscle as it softens and relaxes. Press lightly for pregnant women.
Benefits: Aids circulation, relieves uptightness, irritability, fatigue, shoulder tension, cold hands and feet, headaches.

Arm Circulation: Point #6

Location: Two-thirds up from the back of the armpit crease to the outer shoulder bone.
Finger Application: Press directly on the muscular cord in the shoulder joint, angling the pressure in toward the heart.

Benefits: Aids circulation, relieves hypertension, arm problems (pain, tingling, numbness, cold hands, pain or pressure in the shoulder blades, stiff neck, shoulder tension.

Hand Circulation: Point #3

Location: On the hairy or tanned side of the forearm, two finger-widths from the wrist crease, midway between the two forearm bones.
Finger Application: Firmly press between the bones on the outside of the forearm. This is the Master Point of Great Regulator Channel.
Benefits: Aids circulation, also relieves rheumatism, shoulder and neck pain, temporal headaches, influenza, cold, fatigue, fear, wrist, and weak or trembling fingers .

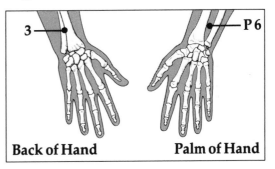

Back of Hand   Palm of Hand

Hand Circulation Point: P 6

Location: On the inside of the forearm, two finger-widths from the wrist crease, midway between the two forearm bones.
Finger Application: Firmly press between the radius and ulna, one or two inches above the wrist. Press lightly for pregnant women.
Benefits: Aids circulation, relieves nausea, insomnia, emotional imbalances,

irregular menstrual periods, diarrhea, dizziness, epilepsy, difficult breathing.

Leg Circulation Points: Sp 12, Sp 13
Location: In the middle of the groin crease where the leg joins the trunk of the body on a vertical line up from the midline of the thigh.

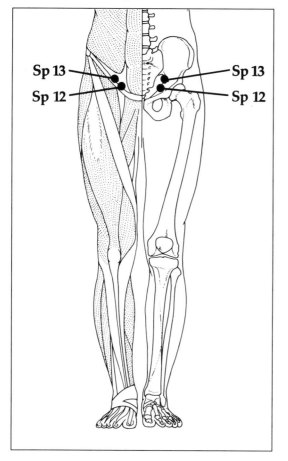

Benefits: Aids circulation, relieves pelvic tension, groin pain, menstrual tension, stomach discomforts, indigestion, cold feet, frustration, sexual tension, and imbalances.

Foot Circulation Point: Sp 4
Location: On the upper arch of the foot, one thumb-width away from the ball of the foot toward the heel.

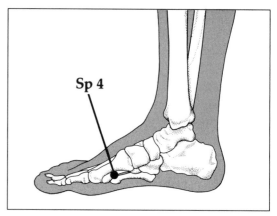

Finger Application: Firmly press into the muscle that runs over the foot arch.
Benefits: Aids circulation, relieves indigestion, stomachaches, hypochondria, worry, foot cramps, and cold feet.

Finger Application: Lean into the groin with the heel of the hand or use your fingers to gradually press inward.

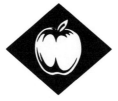

CHAPTER VIII

DIETARY
CONSIDERATIONS

DIETARY CONSIDERATIONS

We have dealt so far with self-massage and stretching to relieve arthritic pain, but there are many contributing causes of arthritis. Diet, of course, is one important factor. What we eat and how much we eat of various foods can affect an arthritic condition. It is important to know which foods to eliminate, which to avoid, and which to emphasize, not only for managing arthritic pain, but also for benefiting the overall condition of our health.

In this chapter, we will examine various dietary principles and practical dietary considerations. We will cover which foods aggravate an arthritic condition and which foods are beneficial for preventing arthritis. We will also discuss the various minerals and vitamins that have been used and tested by doctors who have taken a holistic approach to helping their patients with arthritis.

There are numerous dietary options and a large spectrum of choices on the right way to eat. As individuals, we all have different nutritional needs. Every person has a unique combination of past eating habits, tastes, parental influences, climate, lifestyle, physical activity, and metabolism.

A healthy, balanced diet can be considered the body's most basic medicine. We are what we eat. If we eat highly processed foods, the internal organs responsible for breaking down, digesting, assimilating and eliminating material become sluggish. As a result, the entire digestive system gets congested. Over the years, this can affect the circulation and the condition of the joints. Below is a collection of various specific dietary recommendations for alleviating arthritis. The more we eat natural, unprocessed, whole foods and learn how to balance our diet and exercise as well, the better our health will be.

> ...There is overwhelming evidence that nutritionally balanced meals eaten regularly benefit anyone's overall health, muscle tone, and in the case of arthritis, build the ability to resist the wear and tear of the disease.[42]

> Chinese herbalists advise sufferers of rheumatism and arthritis to avoid greasy foods, bread, pork, white sugar, white flour products and acidity fruits.[43]

> Arthritis is caused by excessive consumption of extremely unbalanced

---

[42] The Arthritis Foundation, *Diet and Arthritis — A Handbook for Patients*, 1987.

[43] Richard Lucas, *Secrets of the Chinese Herbalists*, Cornerstone Library, 1977, p. 104.

foods such as meat and sugar, over a long period of time. This is a lack of good quality fats and a chronic acid condition in the blood. The most important theory is to stop eating 'extreme' kinds of foods. Citrus fruits should be avoided.[44]

Of the vegetables, potatoes, cabbage, green peppers, and all the leafy greens are rich in the vitamins and minerals valuable to the arthritic. Brussels sprouts, beets, peas, beans, carrots and celery are all very good.[45]

Dr. Collin Dong, a graduate of Stanford University Medical School, who at age thirty-five was afflicted with arthritis, helped himself with a particular diet basically consisting of rice, fish, and plenty of vegetables. Dr. Dong recommends eating seafood, vegetables, avocados, sunflower seeds, nuts, safflower oil, rice, soybean products, parsley, onions, garlic, whole grain bread, egg whites, margarine (free of milk solids, such as Mazola) and honey. He further recommends avoiding meat, tomatoes, dairy products, chocolate, dry roasted nuts, soft drinks, alcoholic beverages, and all additives, especially MSG.

The best way to know the right diet for you is to experiment with and inform yourself about a variety of ways of eating.[46] Experience for yourself what effect different diets have on your arthritis or rheumatism. Try different foods, quantities, combinations, and ratios. This way, you can learn firsthand what diet makes you feel best. Remember, however, that

the "ideal diet" can change! As the seasons change, our dietary needs change also.[47]

When you do alter your diet, remember to use moderation, since extreme changes tend to cause imbalances. Results do not usually occur overnight, although you may experience some immediate effects. Benefits from these dietary changes will occur gradually; be patient and give your body time to adjust.

Minerals and Vitamins

Many doctors use minerals and vitamins to help their patients relieve and prevent arthritic pain. It is essential to have periodic urine and blood tests to monitor your system's responses to specific minerals and vitamins. Calcium, along with the vitamin B complex and vitamins C and E have been found particularly important for the prevention and relief of arthritis and rheumatism.[48]

---

[44] Naboru Muramoto, *Healing Ourselves*, Avon Books, 1973, p. 118.

[45] Collin H. Dong, M.D., and Jane Bank, *The Arthritis Cookbook*, Bantam Books, 1973, p. 29.

[46] Naboru Muramoto, *Healing Ourselves*, Avon Books, 1973. A great book on Oriental dietary therapy.

[47] Elson M. Hass, M.D., *Staying Healthy with the Seasons*, Celestial Arts, 1981. A highly recommended book on health and nutrition in relation to seasonal changes.

[48] Irna and Laurence Gadd, *Arthritis Alternatives*, Warner Books, 1965, pp. 86-88.

Calcium

Suffers of arthritic pain have often been found to have a calcium deficiency.[49]

Dr. L. W. Cromwell of San Diego, California, reported to the Gerontological Society of San Francisco that he had found calcium deficiency to be a cause of arthritic crippling. This deficiency, he said, leads first to osteoporosis (loss of bone substance). Then, owing to depletion of bone calcium, the body compensates by depositing extra calcium at the points of greatest stress — the joints — which gives rise to increased rigidity at the joints.[50]

The need for calcium increases as we get older. Aging tends to have an absorbing effect on the body's ability to assimilate calcium. As we get older, the body tends to have greater difficulty assimilating calcium, and its need for calcium also increases. Although the U.S. government suggested a minimum daily requirement for calcium of 800 mg., it must be taken with vitamins A, C, and D, as well as phosphorous and magnesium. Sesame seeds, fish, kelp, and leafy green vegetables are naturally high in these minerals and vitamins.

The following minerals and vitamins help the system to absorb calcium:
- Phosphorous
- Magnesium
- Vitamins A, C, and D

It is important to eat natural foods that have these substances. The minerals and vitamins contained in these foods enable the proper absorption of calcium:
- Parsley
- Wheat Germ
- Raw Sunflower Seeds
- Tofu

Vitamin B Complex

Studies have shown that B vitamins are useful (up to 1,000 mg. per day) for relieving arthritic[51] and rheumatic pains.[52] Vitamin B complex has been found to be important for restoring and nourishing the nervous system. In rheumatism, the nerve sheaths become inflamed. By regularly eating whole grains, seeds, tofu, leafy vegetables, and other foods high in the vitamin B complex, you can often substantially decrease the pain associated with rheumatism and arthritis.

Vitamin E

Vitamin E helps the blood circulate through the joints and muscles. Therefore, vitamin E can be a helpful factor or agent for relieving arthritic and rheumatic pain.

An Israeli study, published in the *Journal of the American Geriatrics Society* (July 1978), reported that 50 percent of patients taking daily dosages of 600 international units of vitamin E had "marked relief from pain."[53]

---

[49] Irna and Laurence Gadd, *Arthritis Alternatives*, Warner Books, 1965, pp. 86-88.

[50] Leonard Mervyn, *Rheumatism and Arthritis*, Thorsons Publishing Group, 1986, p. 76.

[51] Leonard Mervyn, *Rheumatism and Arthritis*, Thorsons Publishing Group, 1986, pp. 71-72.

[52] Irna and Laurence Gadd, *Arthritis Alternatives*, Warner Books, 1965, p. 87.

[53] Irna and Laurence Gadd, *Arthritis Alternatives*, Warner Books, 1965, p. 86.

Considerable investigation in vitamin E has been carried out in the Arthritis Clinic, Rochester General Hospital, Rochester, N.Y., by Dr. C. L. Steinberg. Reporting in the Annals of the New York Academy of Science, he states that he gave vitamin E to 300 patients and relief from pain was obtained in the vast majority of cases. He recommended patients to keep on with a 'maintenance' dose after the symptoms have gone.[54]

Special Foods and Recipes

Miso is a dark paste made from an aged mixture of soybeans and salt. It is used to make soups, sauces, and dips. This common Oriental food is widely used in traditional dietary therapy to soothe arthritis.

Do not salt your food when you use miso, since it already has salt in it. Use about a level teaspoon for a bowl of soup. Since boiling miso destroys its nutrients and digestive enzymes, always add the miso paste after cooking.

Miso helps to restore the beneficial intestinal bacteria and aids in the digestion and assimilation of food. Miso also generally strengthens the metabolism and alkalizes the system, which is good for anemic and arthritic people.[55]

Here's a recipe I recommend:

Miso Soup
(Serves six)

1 tbsp sesame oil
2 celery stalks
2 large onions, diced
5 tomatoes
4 cloves minced garlic
2 large carrots
$1/4$ tsp basil
1 cup fresh broccoli
dash of pepper to taste
2 medium zucchinis
2 tbsp miso paste

Heat the sesame oil in a large kettle. Add the onions, celery, and garlic. Saute with spices for five minutes. Add all the chopped vegetables and cover with 6 cups of water or vegetable or chicken broth. Simmer for ten minutes. Turn off the heat. Dilute miso with several table-spoons of hot broth, and add to the soup. Do not boil the miso. Stir well and serve immediately.

I have found the following recipes helpful for arthritis patients. These recipes have been formulated with special ingredients that contain minerals and vitamins that naturally fortify the body, especially for those with arthritic conditions. When you consistently eat these special foods a couple of times a week, you will become more healthy and feel better too.

[54] Leonard Mervyn, *Rheumatism and Arthritis,* Thorsons Publishing Group, 1986, p. 73.
[55] Naboru Muramoto, *Healing Ourselves,* Avon Books, 1973, p. 83.

Crisp Nut Salad
(Serves four to six)

Soak one cup of raw, whole almonds or raw peanuts overnight. Then drain, rinse and cover with fresh water. Refrigerate the nuts. Dice the following vegetables:

3 stalks of celery
2 to 3 green onions
2 carrots
1 bunch parsley
1 cup cabbage
1 cup fresh lettuce

Drain the nuts and mix together with the vegetables. Make the following light, tasty sauce, or use your favorite salad dressing.

2 tbsp soy sauce or tamari
2 tbsp lemon juice or rice vinegar
2 tbsp sesame oil or sweet almond oil
dash of pepper to taste
dash of onion or garlic powder

Toss the salad with the dressing, top with wheat germ and/or lightly toasted sesame seeds and serve.

Kombu

This variety of seaweed is traditionally believed to be very good for arthritis, high and low blood pressure, and tumors. Soak and cook along with vegetables.

Grilled Rice

Dry roast raw brown rice in a cast iron frying pan under medium heat for fifteen to twenty minutes until well-browned. Eat small amounts, chewing very thoroughly, twice a day without boiling. In traditional Chinese dietary therapy, this rice is good for hyper-insulinism and rheumatism.

Dandelion Root

Sauté small pieces. Add a little tamari and cook a little longer. This is traditionally believed to be good for arthritis, cardiac problems, and rheumatism.

Traditional Chinese doctors advise sufferers of rheumatism and arthritis to avoid acid-forming foods such as baked goods, dairy products (especially hard cheeses), pork, white sugar, white flour products, and acidic fruits. Meals should include steamed vegetables, unpolished brown rice, or alkaline fruits. People with gout should avoid alcoholic beverages, especially beer. Rich, starchy foods are especially forbidden.

The ancient Chinese herbalists discovered that *Fo-Ti-Tieng Roots Tea* (available at better health food stores) effectively dissolves toxic build-up in the body and joints. It is therefore used as an anti-inflammatory remedy for relieving bursitis, rheumatism, arthritis, and gout.

Celery is used in China not only as a food, but also as a remedy for the relief of neuralgia, nervousness, rheumatism, arthritis, gout, and lumbago. A strong tea made from celery seeds, along with plenty of celery in the diet, can help to neutralize uric acids in the body.

Celery Tea

Place three tablespoons of celery seeds in two quarts of water. Cover the container and allow to simmer slowly for three hours. Then strain. Drink one cup of hot tea three or four times daily.

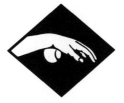

CHAPTER IX

SELF-HELP
TOOLS

SELF-HELP TOOLS

This chapter will give you some additional Arthritis Relief ideas using common objects as self-help tools. Although your fingertips are one of the strongest yet sensitive healing tools that you have, it is important not to be dependent solely on using your fingers to relieve pressure or pain, especially if they have been weakened by arthritis.

The following pages will cover tools that you can make yourself with common household items. For other resources, such as video and audio cassette tapes, charts, and natural pain-relief products, contact the Acupressure Institute.[56] At the end of this chapter you will find suggestions for using mental techniques — namely, affirmations and visualizations — to relieve arthritic pain. I offer to you these resources and suggestions in the hope that you will be encouraged to take your health into your own hands.

Golf Balls

The size and shape of a golf ball makes it an especially useful tool for massaging and exercising arthritic joints.

---

[56] Request the Acupressure Institute's free products and book catalog. Be sure to mention that you are interested in Arthritis Relief self-help tools. Acupressure Institute, 1533 Shattuck Avenue, Berkeley, California 94709. Tel. (415) 845-1059, 1-800-442-2232 outside California only.

It is often helpful to keep a couple of golf balls at work and at home in convenient places, such as nearby the chair or couch where you watch television, in your purse or coat pocket, on the night stand beside your bed, in the glove compartment of your car, or by the telephone.

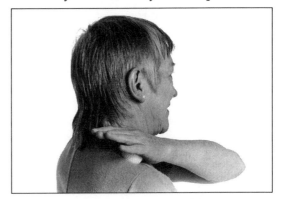

Massage: Golf balls can enable you to massage yourself without straining your hands. Place the ball in the palm of your hand and roll it over the area to be massaged. Experiment with different movements and tempos, such as small, rapid, circular movements compared to large, slow, back and forth movements.

Foot Massage: Place a golf ball on the floor while you are sitting comfortably in a straight-back chair. With the bottom of your foot on the golf ball, slowly roll it to massage the bottom of your foot, stimulating the reflexology points. If you find a sore spot, hold it steady with lighter pressure without moving the ball for a minute or two, and breathe deeply.

You can also use two golf balls simultaneously, one for each foot, while you are at your desk, talking on the telephone, or watching television. The golf ball foot massage can be done either barefooted or while wearing socks.

Hand Arthritis: The golf ball is an excellent tool for massaging and exercising arthritic joints in the hands.[57] Slowly roll the ball between your hands to stimulate all areas on the palm and the outside of the hand between the bones.

You can also use two golf balls to exercise your hands for preventing and relieving arthritic pain. With the palm facing up, place two golf balls in the palm of that hand. Slowly and gracefully roll the two balls around as you move your hand. It is helpful to time yourself as you do this hand exercise. It is important to slowly increase the amount of time you spend, being careful not to overstrain, especially if you have rheumatoid arthritis.

Clothespins

Foot and Hand Pain: There are acupressure points at the base of each nail that can help relieve pain in the fingers and toes. If you ever have a pain that extends down into your fingers or toes, you will be able to relieve it by putting firm pressure on the digital nerves that are close to the base of the nail.

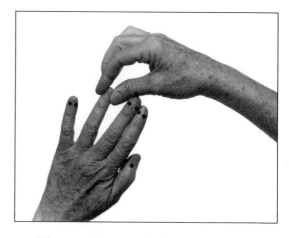

These points need about two or three minutes of firm, prolonged pressure. You can use your thumb and index finger to hold both sides at the base of the nails of the fingers or toes. Often your fingers will become tired of holding that long. Try using a clothespin to hold these points instead of your fingers. Wrap a washcloth or a small cotton rag around the finger or toe on which you want to work. Then apply the clothespin(s) to the base of the nail(s). Adjust the clothespin as comfortably as you can. After a minute or two, you can remove the clothespin(s) and use your hands normally.

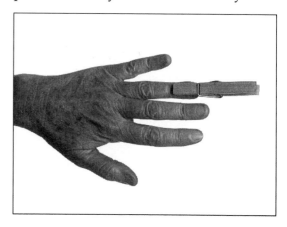

---

[57] *Note:* Please refer to the chapter on hands (pages 69-106) for more specific techniques that utilize golf balls.

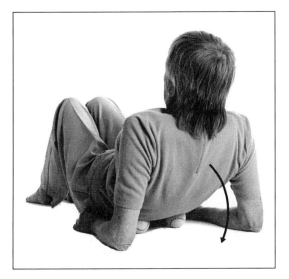

Tennis Balls

Back Massage: Tennis balls or small rubber balls can be helpful for massaging the hard-to-reach areas on your back. Place a couple of balls close together on a carpeted floor. Sit down on the rug with the balls in back of you, your knees bent, and feet flat on the floor in front of you. Slowly lean back on your elbow, gradually reclining and placing the balls beneath the part of your back that needs to be massaged.

Once you roll the balls onto the desired spot, hold that position as you take several long, slow, deep breaths with your head relaxed backward. Then gradually roll the balls onto another tense area. Hold that position for a minute while you take several more deep breaths with your eyes closed.

After you have relieved most of your back tension, put the balls aside and lie down on your back with your eyes closed. Completely relax for about five minutes, taking slow, deep breaths.

Hands and Wrists: Place a tennis ball on a table. Cover the ball with the palm of your hand, moving it in small, slow, circular motions. Roll the tennis ball slowly between your fingers to stretch them. Then move the ball underneath the inside of your wrist crease, making slow circular motions to massage the wrist joint. Gradually work your way up your forearm. Then switch to work on your opposite hand.

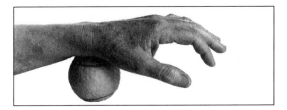

Place your left hand on the table with the palm facing down. Holding the tennis ball in your right hand, place the ball on top of your left hand and slowly roll it in between the bones (metacarpal) over the top of your left hand. After rolling the ball between each finger, switch sides to massage the top of your right hand.

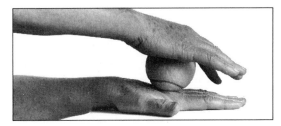

Strengthening the Hands: Grasp the tennis ball in your left hand and gently squeeze it five times. Then grasp the ball in your right hand and squeeze it five times. Gradually increase the number of times you squeeze the ball to strengthen the joints in your hands and fingers.

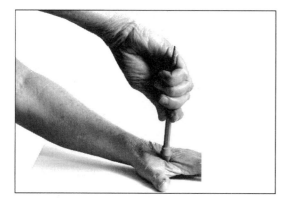

Pencil Eraser

Since many people have difficulty pressing some of the points for prolonged time periods (due to weakness, arthritic degeneration, or pain in the hands), the tip of a pencil eraser can be a helpful tool. The length of a pencil should be long enough to easily grasp, since it will become a handle. The eraser should not be too short since it will be the probe that you will use for applying the pressure. Use the pencil eraser to press any acupressure points that are difficult for you to do using your fingers, e.g., feet, legs, arms, hands, etc.

Avocado Pit

An avocado pit can be used similarly to a golf ball since it is approximately the same size. One advantage of the avocado pit is that it has a more pointed surface that you can carefully use to get into hard-to-get-at areas. This makes it an excellent tool for massaging the acupressure points in the hands and feet, especially in the joints. Use the avocado pit in these areas, gently holding the points for two to three minutes, repeating this two or three times daily.

The avocado pit can also be used to massage the foot reflexology points on the bottoms of the feet. Just like the golf balls, place the avocado pit on the ground with the bottom of your foot over it as you roll onto various foot reflex points.

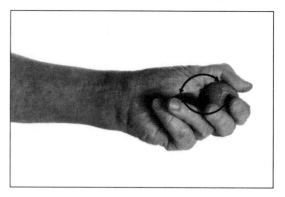

You can also use the avocado pit in the palm of your hand to massage any area of your body. If you have two avocado pits, you can hold them together in one hand (with your palm facing up) and slowly rotate them as you move your fingers to exercise your hands. If you have rheumatoid arthritis, this exercise should be practiced in moderation along with substantial periods of deep relaxation not only for your hands, but for the rest of your body as well. Rotating two pits in one hand is an excellent medicinal exercise for osteoarthritis in the hands.

A Towel
Making Your Own Custom Back Roller
Materials:
- One-inch thick round wooden dowel or rubber tube, about 12 inches in length
- One large, thick towel
- Two pieces of heavy string or ribbon (2 feet each)

Instructions:

1. Lay the towel out flat. Fold the outer edges in toward the center, as shown.

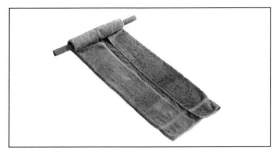

2. Place the dowel or tube at one end of the towel. Roll the towel up around the dowel.
3. Tie string or rope around the towel to hold it in place.
4. Place your roller on the ground. Lie down on your back with the roller underneath you.

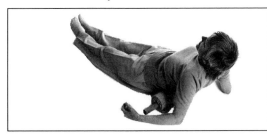

5. Roll it to an area of your back that feels tense or sore.

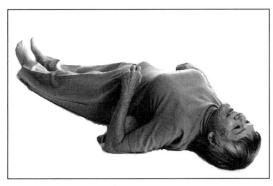

6. Stay on that area for about a minute with your eyes closed, breathing deeply and slowly.
7. Move the roller to other tense areas of your back and repeat #6.

Bringing your knees toward your abdomen will increase the pressure of the roller on your lower back. Breathe in as you bring your legs up, and breathe out as you slowly pull your knees toward your chest. Continue to breathe deeply as you hold your knees in a comfortable position.[58]

Neck Stretches

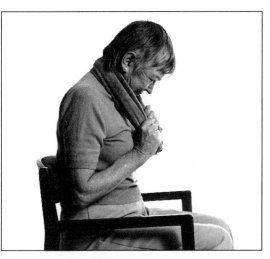

Sit comfortably in a chair. Drape a medium-size towel over your neck with the ends of the towel hanging over your chest. Grasp the ends of the towel firmly, with your head relaxed forward. Apply

[58] *Note:* You can further customize this back roller by using two tennis or golf balls instead of the tube. Place the balls about three inches apart and roll the towel up around the two balls.

firm pressure downward to stretch your neck for five to ten seconds. Take a long, deep breath as you bring your head upward. Exhale as you apply the pressure for five to ten seconds. Continue the exercise several more times to relieve tension in your shoulders and neck.

Leg Stretches

Sit on a carpeted floor with your legs extended straight out in front of you. Place the center of a large towel around the bottom of your feet and grasp hold of the ends of the towel. Inhale as you stretch up, straightening your back. Exhale as you pull down with your arm muscles, bringing your forehead down toward your knees and keeping your knees straight. Inhale up and exhale down, continuing the exercise several more times.

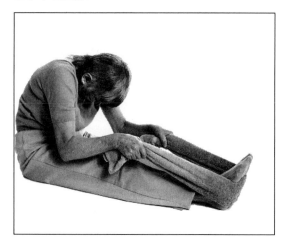

Benefits: This exercise stretches the "life nerve" (sciatic nerve), one of the largest nerves of the body. Gently stretching this nerve daily is an important key to promoting a longer and healthier life.

Warm-Hot Water

Baths, hot tubs, saunas, jacuzzis, and hot compresses are important for relieving arthritic pain. Increased effectiveness is the result of combining regular daily heat application, along with the therapeutic exercises contained in this book.

The ritual of taking baths can be an important part of your arthritis relief program. Try preparing your bath with different essential oils, such as eucalyptus or oil of mint (available in drug and health food stores). Epson salts can be another soothing addition to your bath. While bathing, do some of the self-care exercises in this book or try doing the morning or afternoon daily routines in a warm room immediately after taking your bath. Then lie down on your back and let yourself completely relax.

Also treat yourself to regular foot baths and foot massages. Be sure to take regular hand baths as well. It is highly beneficial to massage your hands under the flow of warm-hot water in the sink for a few minutes, several times a day. Move your hands over one another as if you are washing them with soap. The combination of the movement with the hot water and deep breathing is great for arthritic joints.

Showers can also be highly therapeutic to massage the whole body. It is important to have a shower head that will massage your body firmly with a strong water pressure. You can easily purchase a shower massage head unit at any hardware store. Feel free to experiment with different ways to stretch your body and massage yourself while in the shower.

The combination of the hot water with the stimulation of self-massage and stretching results in increased benefits.

EXTERNAL TREATMENTS

Soya Plaster

Soak one cup of soya beans in five cups of water for 24 hours. Crush and add 10 percent wheat flour. Apply to the forehead for fever or to any inflamed area. It absorbs fever and inflammations of arthritic spots on the body.

Ginger Compresses

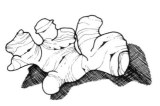

A hot ginger compress is effective for releasing muscular tension and stiff, aching arthritic joints.[59] Grate four ounces raw ginger. Place it in cheese cloth or into a cotton sack. Bring $1/2$ gallon water to a boil. Turn off flame. Drop the sack into the water. When water turns pale yellow, dip a towel in it. Ring out the excess water and cover the area with the hot towel. Cover compress with another towel to prevent rapid cooling. The water temperature should be as hot as you can tolerate without burning the skin. Redip the towel when it cools. Continue for 15 minutes or until the skin becomes pinkish.

[59] *Note:* If your joints feel hot, swollen, and reddish, do not apply these hot compresses. See your doctor for a medical opinion.

Benefits: Ginger compresses are especially effective for relieving arthritic aches and pains as well as for releasing chronic muscular tension in the back. Apply compresses directly on these tense, stiff areas.

Ginger Bath

Slice one pound fresh ginger into small pieces. Place in cotton sack or tie up in some cheese cloth and boil in two gallons of water for one hour. Dump this water in a hot bath and soak until the water begins to cool. This is especially good for leg, ankle, knee and hip pains as well as lower backaches.

Tofu Plaster

Use a cheese cloth to squeeze the liquid out of tofu. Mix the tofu with about 10 percent wheat flour to further dry it out and hold it together. Spread this directly on an area that is painful or inflamed. This is good for relieving arthritic inflammation and hot, feverish areas.

Hops

Traditionally, hops have been used to bring relief from the pain of neuralgia, sciatica, arthritis, rheumatism, and lumbago. A poultice is made by putting a handful of hops in a muslin bag and tying the bag securely, but leaving enough room for the hops to swell. The bag is placed in a container of hot water for a few minutes, then wrung out and applied to the painful area as hot as possible. Cover with a dry towel to retain the heat.

Mugwort Leaves

Steam the leaves and apply as a poultice for the relief of aches and pains.

Rosemary

This herb was brought from Rome to China during the Wei dynasty. Oil of rosemary and oil of juniper mixed together in equal amounts is used for the relief of arthritic joints and is especially good for backaches.

Peanut Oil

After warming, use this oil for massage to reduce joint inflammation and pain of arthritis. The joints are massaged three times a day. This remedy works slowly, but is said to bring good results.

Camphor

When mixed with Chinese wine, camphor is used as a liniment for muscular aches and pains.

AFFIRMATION AND VISUALIZATION FOR PAIN RELIEF

As you take a few long, deep breaths, think of the positive qualities you have now and can draw on for the rest of your life. Tell yourself:

I am going to give myself whatever it takes to relieve and heal my arthritis. I have faith that I will be given all that I need to become healthier. I trust that I will make decisions to create a lifestyle that enriches my health.

Now visualize yourself driving a chariot, firmly holding the reins that govern your creativity and potential in life. Take a few slow, long, deep breaths while you envision and clarify your greatest challenges and aspirations. As you continue to breathe deeply, visualize yourself taking hold of the reins of your life, with trust, courage, conviction, and a clear vision for making wise, healthy decisions along the way.

The following affirmation will help you become familiar with that strong, righteous, wise chariot. Take some deep breaths while you say to yourself:

The decisions that I make for relieving my arthritis are wise, helpful, sound decisions. I am constantly being guided by the awareness of my body. I inspire myself moment to moment by taking deep inspiration. I know that I am taking the necessary steps to create a pain-free, healthy life.

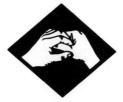

CHAPTER X

ARTHRITIS
ACCOUNT
DIARY

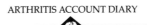

ARTHRITIS ACCOUNT DIARY

Use the following pages weekly to record changes, activities, and events as you work to relieve and improve your arthritic condition. A personal record of your exercise program and the process of physical change that results can be valuable information. This diary can make you more conscious of changes that occur over a period of time and can serve as a source of inspiration for continuing to take your health into your own hands.

Your weekly account will tell you:

❑ Where your pain focuses and radiates;

❑ When your arthritis hurts the most;

❑ What causes your health problems;

❑ What makes your pain worse;

❑ Which techniques help relieve the pain;

❑ How much progress you have made over a period of time.

KEEPING AN ACCOUNT OF MY PROGRESS

Date: _____

Present condition is:

❏ painful ❏ tense
❏ stiff ❏ aching
❏ tired

The pain is:

❏ sharp ❏ off and on
❏ dull ❏ steady

When my arthritis hurts the most:

Time of day: _____

❏ after sleeping
❏ during work
❏ before sleeping

Where my pain is centered:

Use the drawing provided below. Mark in one color the area of most discomfort. Then use another color to show where the pain travels in the body and to specify other areas of tension, pain, or stiffness.

❏ knees ❏ into the upper back
❏ elbows ❏ into the lower back
❏ legs ❏ into the neck
❏ arms ❏ through the ribs
❏ feet ❏ down the back of the leg
❏ wrists ❏ along the side of the leg
❏ toes ❏ into the hips
❏ hands ❏ across the back
❏ fingers

Which fingers or toes? _____

_____

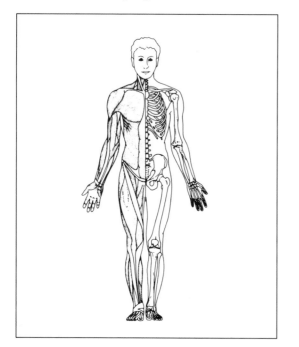

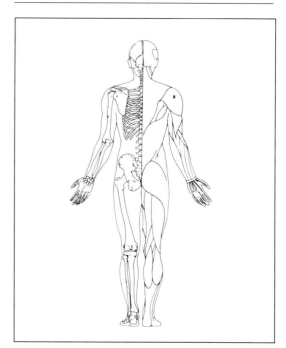

What makes my arthritis worse?

- ❑ standing
- ❑ cold weather
- ❑ sitting
- ❑ menstruation
- ❑ bending over
- ❑ stress
- ❑ lifting
- ❑ constipation
- ❑ driving
- ❑ pressure from: _____

My arthritis has affected my:

- ❑ sleep
- ❑ appetite
- ❑ breathing
- ❑ elimination
- ❑ work
- ❑ outlook on life
- ❑ relationships

What has helped to relieve my pain?

- ❑ massage
- ❑ sleep
- ❑ meditation
- ❑ acupressure points
- ❑ exercise _____
  (specify kind, e.g., swimming)

My Arthritis Relief practice:

Choose four techniques or exercises from this book that have helped to relieve your arthritis.

1. _____ on page ____

2. _____ on page ____

3. _____ on page ____

4. _____ on page ____

Results: Describe the changes that have occurred.

_____
_____
_____
_____
_____
_____
_____
_____
_____
_____
_____
_____

KEEPING AN ACCOUNT OF MY PROGRESS

Date: _____

Present condition is:

❑ painful ❑ tense
❑ stiff ❑ aching
❑ tired

The pain is:

❑ sharp ❑ off and on
❑ dull ❑ steady

When my arthritis hurts the most:

Time of day: _____

❑ after sleeping
❑ during work
❑ before sleeping

Where my pain is centered:

Use the drawing provided below. Mark in one color the area of most discomfort. Then use another color to show where the pain travels in the body and to specify other areas of tension, pain, or stiffness.

❑ knees ❑ into the upper back
❑ elbows ❑ into the lower back
❑ legs ❑ into the neck
❑ arms ❑ through the ribs
❑ feet ❑ down the back of the leg
❑ wrists ❑ along the side of the leg
❑ toes ❑ into the hips
❑ hands ❑ across the back
❑ fingers

Which fingers or toes? _____

_____

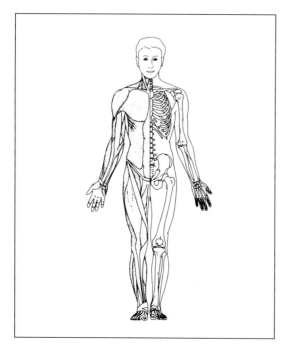

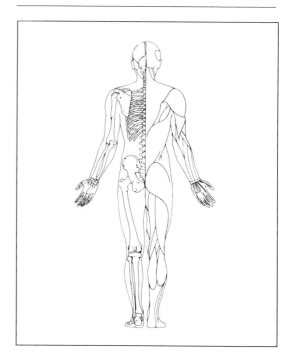

What makes my arthritis worse?

- ❏ standing
- ❏ cold weather
- ❏ sitting
- ❏ menstruation
- ❏ bending over
- ❏ stress
- ❏ lifting
- ❏ constipation
- ❏ driving
- ❏ pressure from: _____

My arthritis has affected my:

- ❏ sleep
- ❏ appetite
- ❏ breathing
- ❏ elimination
- ❏ work
- ❏ outlook on life
- ❏ relationships

What has helped to relieve my pain?

- ❏ massage
- ❏ sleep
- ❏ meditation
- ❏ acupressure points
- ❏ exercise _____
  (specify kind, e.g., swimming)

My Arthritis Relief practice:

Choose four techniques or exercises from this book that have helped to relieve your arthritis.

1. _____ on page _____

2. _____ on page _____

3. _____ on page _____

4. _____ on page _____

Results: Describe the changes that have occurred.

_____

_____

_____

_____

_____

_____

_____

_____

_____

_____

_____

KEEPING AN ACCOUNT OF MY PROGRESS

Date: _____

Present condition is:

- ❏ painful   ❏ tense
- ❏ stiff   ❏ aching
- ❏ tired

The pain is:

- ❏ sharp   ❏ off and on
- ❏ dull   ❏ steady

When my arthritis hurts the most:

Time of day: _____

- ❏ after sleeping
- ❏ during work
- ❏ before sleeping

Where my pain is centered:

Use the drawing provided below. Mark in one color the area of most discomfort. Then use another color to show where the pain travels in the body and to specify other areas of tension, pain, or stiffness.

- ❏ knees   ❏ into the upper back
- ❏ elbows   ❏ into the lower back
- ❏ legs   ❏ into the neck
- ❏ arms   ❏ through the ribs
- ❏ feet   ❏ down the back of the leg
- ❏ wrists   ❏ along the side of the leg
- ❏ toes   ❏ into the hips
- ❏ hands   ❏ across the back
- ❏ fingers

Which fingers or toes? _____

_____

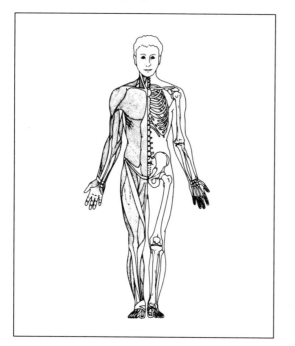

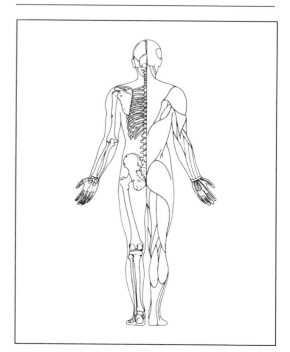

What makes my arthritis worse?

❑ standing
❑ cold weather
❑ sitting
❑ menstruation
❑ bending over
❑ stress
❑ lifting
❑ constipation
❑ driving
❑ pressure from: _____

My arthritis has affected my:

❑ sleep
❑ appetite
❑ breathing
❑ elimination
❑ work
❑ outlook on life
❑ relationships

What has helped to relieve my pain?

❑ massage
❑ sleep
❑ meditation
❑ acupressure points
❑ exercise _____
  (specify kind, e.g., swimming)

My Arthritis Relief practice:

Choose four techniques or exercises from this book that have helped to relieve your arthritis.

1. _____ on page _____

2. _____ on page _____

3. _____ on page _____

4. _____ on page _____

Results: Describe the changes that have occurred.

_____

_____

_____

_____

_____

_____

_____

_____

_____

_____

_____

_____

KEEPING AN ACCOUNT OF MY PROGRESS

Date: _____

Present condition is:

❏ painful ❏ tense
❏ stiff ❏ aching
❏ tired

The pain is:

❏ sharp ❏ off and on
❏ dull ❏ steady

When my arthritis hurts the most:

Time of day: _____

❏ after sleeping
❏ during work
❏ before sleeping

Where my pain is centered:

Use the drawing provided below. Mark in one color the area of most discomfort. Then use another color to show where the pain travels in the body and to specify other areas of tension, pain, or stiffness.

❏ knees ❏ into the upper back
❏ elbows ❏ into the lower back
❏ legs ❏ into the neck
❏ arms ❏ through the ribs
❏ feet ❏ down the back of the leg
❏ wrists ❏ along the side of the leg
❏ toes ❏ into the hips
❏ hands ❏ across the back
❏ fingers

Which fingers or toes? _____

_____

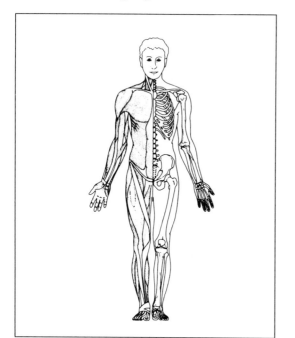
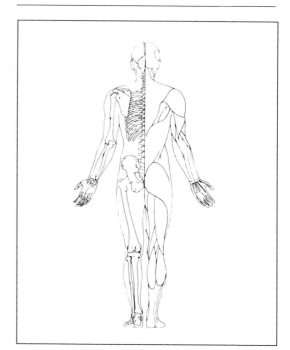

What makes my arthritis worse?

- ❏ standing
- ❏ cold weather
- ❏ sitting
- ❏ menstruation
- ❏ bending over
- ❏ stress
- ❏ lifting
- ❏ constipation
- ❏ driving
- ❏ pressure from: _____

My arthritis has affected my:

- ❏ sleep
- ❏ appetite
- ❏ breathing
- ❏ elimination
- ❏ work
- ❏ outlook on life
- ❏ relationships

What has helped to relieve my pain?

- ❏ massage
- ❏ sleep
- ❏ meditation
- ❏ acupressure points
- ❏ exercise _____
  (specify kind, e.g., swimming)

My Arthritis Relief practice:

Choose four techniques or exercises from this book that have helped to relieve your arthritis.

1. _____ on page _____

2. _____ on page _____

3. _____ on page _____

4. _____ on page _____

Results: Describe the changes that have occurred.

_____

_____

_____

_____

_____

_____

_____

_____

_____

_____

_____

_____

_____

KEEPING AN ACCOUNT OF MY PROGRESS

Date: _____

Present condition is:

❑ painful   ❑ tense
❑ stiff   ❑ aching
❑ tired

The pain is:

❑ sharp   ❑ off and on
❑ dull   ❑ steady

When my arthritis hurts the most:

Time of day: _____

❑ after sleeping
❑ during work
❑ before sleeping

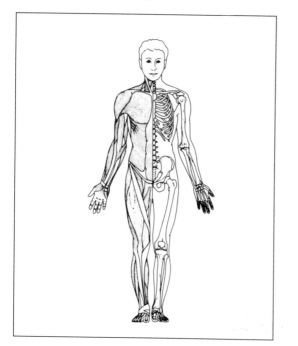

Where my pain is centered:

Use the drawing provided below. Mark in one color the area of most discomfort. Then use another color to show where the pain travels in the body and to specify other areas of tension, pain, or stiffness.

❑ knees   ❑ into the upper back
❑ elbows   ❑ into the lower back
❑ legs   ❑ into the neck
❑ arms   ❑ through the ribs
❑ feet   ❑ down the back of the leg
❑ wrists   ❑ along the side of the leg
❑ toes   ❑ into the hips
❑ hands   ❑ across the back
❑ fingers

Which fingers or toes? _____

_____

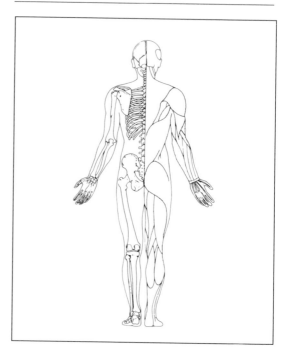

What makes my arthritis worse?

- ❏ standing
- ❏ cold weather
- ❏ sitting
- ❏ menstruation
- ❏ bending over
- ❏ stress
- ❏ lifting
- ❏ constipation
- ❏ driving
- ❏ pressure from: _____

My arthritis has affected my:

- ❏ sleep
- ❏ appetite
- ❏ breathing
- ❏ elimination
- ❏ work
- ❏ outlook on life
- ❏ relationships

What has helped to relieve my pain?

- ❏ massage
- ❏ sleep
- ❏ meditation
- ❏ acupressure points
- ❏ exercise _____
  (specify kind, e.g., swimming)

My Arthritis Relief practice:

Choose four techniques or exercises from this book that have helped to relieve your arthritis.

1. _____ on page ____

2. _____ on page ____

3. _____ on page ____

4. _____ on page ____

Results: Describe the changes that have occurred.

_____

_____

_____

_____

_____

_____

_____

_____

_____

_____

_____

_____

BIBLIOGRAPHY

Academy of Traditional Chinese Medicine. *An Outline of Chinese Acupuncture.* Peking: Foreign Languages Press, 1975.

Airola, Paavo O. *There is a Cure for Arthritis.* New York: Parker Publishing Co., 1968.

Brena, Steven F., M.D. *Yoga and Medicine.* New York: Penguin Books, 1973.

Dong, Collin, M.D. *The Arthritic's Cookbook.* New York: Bantam Books, 1973.

Eisenberg, David, M.D. *Encounters With Qi.* New York: Penguin Books, 1987.

Fries, James, M.D. *Arthritis, A Comprehensive Guide.* Reading, Massachusetts: Addison-Wesley, 1979.

Gach, Michael Reed. *Acu-Yoga: Self Help Techniques.* Tokyo: Japan Publications, 1981.

Gach, Michael Reed. *The Bum Back Book.* Berkeley, California: Celestial Arts, 1983.

Gach, Michael Reed. *Greater Energy At Your Fingertips.* Berkeley, California: Celestial Arts, 1986.

Gadd, Irna and Laurence. *Arthritis Alternatives.* New York: Warner Books, 1985.

Garde, Raghanath K., M.D. *Principles and Practice of Yoga Therapy.* Lakemont, Georgia: Tarnhelm, 1970.

Jackson, Mildred, and Teague, Terri. *The Handbook of Alternatives to Chemical Medicine.* Oakland, California: Lawton-Teague Publications, 1975.

Jayson, Malcolm IV, and Dixon, Allan St. J. *Rheumatism and Arthritis.* London: Pan Books, Ltd., 1980.

Jensen, Bernard. "Arthritis and Rheumatism Pains Are Symptoms." *The Herbalist*, October 1979, 14–16.

Kaptchuk, Ted J. *The Web That Has No Weaver.* New York: Congdon and Weed, 1983.

Leung, Stanley T. W. "The Acupuncture Treatment of Bi Entity." *JACTCM* 3 (1983):34–41.

Lin Jie Hou. "Bi-Entity (Arthritis). Clinical Experience of Master-Physician Wang Wei Lan." *JACTCM* 3 (1983):3–28.

Mann, Felix. *Atlas of Acupuncture.* Philadelphia: International Ideas, 1970.

Masunaga, Shizuto. *Zen Shiatsu.* Tokyo: Japan Publications, 1977.

Mervyn, Leonard, B.S., Ph.D. *Rheumatism and Arthritis.* New York: Thornsons Publishing, 1986.

O'Connor, John. *Acupuncture: A Comprehensive Text.* Edited and translated by Dan Bensky. Seattle: Eastland Press, 1981.

Requena, Yves. *Terrains and Pathology in Acupuncture, Vol. 1.* Massachusetts: Paradigm Publications, 1986.

Revolutionary Health Committee of Hunan Province. *A Barefoot Doctor's Manual.* Seattle: Madrona Publishers, 1977.

Serizawa, Katsusuke, M.D. *Massage: The Oriental Method; Tsubo: Vital Points for Oriental Therapy.* Tokyo: Japan Publications, 1976.

Shealy, Norman, M.D. *The Pain Game,* Berkeley, California: Celestial Arts, 1976.

Siefert, Gary, and Chan, Yimmy, comps. and trans. *Symptom Analysis and Acupuncture.* Sydney: 1984.

Simonton, Carl O., M.D., *Getting Well Again.* New York: Houghton Mifflin Co., 1983.

Teeguarden, Iona. *Acupressure Way of Health.* Tokyo: Japan Publications, 1978.

Terashi, Bohuso. *Chinese Herbal Medicine and the Problems of Aging.* Oriental Healing Arts Institute: 1984.

Todd, Mabel Elsworth. *The Thinking Body.* New York: Dance Horizons Republications, 1975.

Toyohiko, Kikutani. *A Review of the Therapeutic Effect of Fang-Chi-Tang (Staphania and Astragalus Combination)* Oriental Healing Arts Institute: June, 1983.

Van Nghi, Nguyen. *Pathogénie et Pathologie Energétiques en Médecine Chinoise.* Translated by Sydney Acupuncture Study Group. Sydney: 1980.

Veith, Ilza, trans. *The Yellow Emperor's Classic of Internal Medicine.* Berkeley, California: University of California Press, 1949.

Weil, Andrew, M.D., *Health and Healing.* Boston: Houghton Mifflin Co., 1983.

ACUPRESSURE INSTITUTE'S
GIFTS • PRODUCTS • TRAININGS

The Acupressure Institute, founded in 1976 by Michael Reed Gach, was designed to contribute to the welfare of thousands internationally through its stress reduction programs, educational products, workshops, and short intensive programs. The Institute offers comprehensive career training approved by the California Department of Education. A free schedule is available upon request.

Workshops and Trainings

A free school catalog and an application are available upon request.

Workshops for Special Groups

Michael Reed Gach is available to speak and make presentations to local groups of 25 people or more. Write to the Acupressure Institute if you want to sponsor a weekend workshop with Mr. Gach. Choose from the following topics:

- Arthritis Relief

- Acu-Face Lift

- Bum Back Seminar

- Acupressure Weight Loss

- How to Increase Your Vitality

- Releasing Shoulder & Neck Tension

- The Acupressure Sampler
  (Choose four of the above topics)

Learning Tools and Supplies

The Acupressure Institute sells many hard-to-find books and self-acupressure charts, as well as special instructional audio and video tapes. Call or write to receive a free products brochure and order form.

Hawaiian Health Retreats

Each year, Mr. Gach leads an eight-day retreat on tropical Maui, teaching participants how to relieve arthritic pain and stiffness, as well as shoulder and neck tension. You will learn natural breathing exercises and easy stretches, along with acupressure techniques, as you soak up the warmth and beauty of Hawaii. Enrollment is limited to 25. Discounts are available for reservations for two or more people. Send for a free brochure.

Acupressure Institute of America, Inc.
1533 Shattuck Avenue, Dept. 4,
Berkeley, CA 94709

(415) 845-1059 *in California*
1-800-442-2232 *outside California*

GLOSSARY

Abused Joints: Joints that are inflamed by the overuse of nearby muscles, ligaments, or tendons.

Acupressure: An ancient touch therapy that uses the Chinese system of acupuncture points and meridians combined with Japanese finger pressure techniques to release muscular tensions and increase circulation.

Acupuncture: A traditional method of Chinese medicine in which fine needles are inserted into the body in key points to release internal blockages and balance energy.

Acu-Yoga: An integration of acupressure and yoga used for self-treatment.

Adjustment: A chiropractic manipulation to properly align the vertebrae of the spinal column.

Affirmations: Personal statements said aloud or to oneself that validate different aspects of one's existence. They are used to visualize and increase the benefits of Acu-Yoga techniques.

Alignment: Having the spinal vertebrae in proper line.

Alternative Therapies: A wide range of progressive, holistic health techniques not recognized by the majority of Western medicine. The following is a partial list of alternative therapies that have been found effective for relieving arthritis:

Neuro-Muscular Re-Education Techniques: The Alexander Technique and the Feldenkrais Method are the most widely used approaches for retraining the nervous system and neuro-muscular patterns. These gentle methods help to lengthen the muscles and reduce muscular compression and joint pain.

Chiropractic Adjustments: Physical manipulation to properly align the vertebrae of the spinal column.

Yoga Postures: Body positions that stretch and strengthen the spine, limbs, joints, muscles, and nerves to bring about a natural balance of the body and mind.

Tai Chi Chuan: A traditional Chinese system of movement that enables the body to balance and maintain health.

Herbology: The medicinal use of plants for internal and external preparations.

Traditional Chinese Medicine: The ancient Chinese health care system, philosophy, and medical practices as handed down from generation to generation, starting from the first recorded text in 2697 B.C., entitled *The Yellow Emperor's Classic of Internal Medicine.*

Arthritis: Inflammation of the joints. There are over one hundred types of arthritis, most involving pain due to metabolic, infectious, or constitutional causes. It is important to establish a correct diagnosis of the type of arthritis you have. The chapter on The Causes of Arthritis briefly discusses the major types of arthritis, but to get further information on its diagnosis, read *Arthritis, A Comprehensive Guide,* by Dr. James Fries (Reading, Mass.: Addison-Wesley, 1979).

Blockage: An accumulation or congestion of energy in or surrounding an acupressure point. Blockages may ache, be painful, or feel numb before manifesting as a more severe physical symptom.

Breathing Awareness: The ability to deepen and direct the breath into different parts of the body through concentration and relaxation.

Centering: The process of gaining awareness of the mind and body. This enables a person to be more conscious in the present moment.

Cervical Vertebrae: The seven spinal bones of the neck.

Chi: A Chinese word for vital energy. It has been translated as "material energy" or "vital matter" that circulates through the meridians.

Chronic Muscular Tension: A long-term condition in which the muscle fibers are held indefinitely in a shortened, contracted state.

Coccyx: The last vertebra at the base of the spine.

Compresses: The application of heat (sometimes both hot and cold are alternately used) to increase circulation in a particular area.

Deep Relaxation: Letting go of all parts of the body and mind to allow a natural flow of energy to circulate in its natural course. To completely relax after exercise is the best way to recharge the nervous system.

Disease: An imbalance in the system as a whole.

Distal Points: Acupressure points located a distance from the area they benefit. See Local Points.

Energy Blockage: An obstruction to the free flow of vital matter, which manifests physically as tension, pain, or stiffness. Thoughts and emotions can also cause energy blockages.

Frontal Points: Acupressure points located on the front of the body.

Holistic: An approach to life based on a perspective that all forms of existence are unified, that the whole equals more than the sum of its parts, and that every aspect, whether internal or external, affects the whole.

Homeostatis: The state of equilibrium or balance.

Hypertension: Abnormally high arterial blood pressure.

Impotence: The condition of lacking in physical strength and being unable to engage in sexual intercourse.

Jin Shin: A highly developed acupressure massage technique that uses gentle to deep finger pressure applied to specific points on the human anatomy. This system releases tension and rebalances all areas of the body.

Ki: The Japanese word for the vital life energy which concentrates in all living things. It circulates through the human body in pathways called meridians.

Life Force: The vital energy contained in all things. The three main types are:
1. The energy that circulates through the body via the meridians.
2. The power generated from the human qualities of love, devotion, determination, will power, and positive thinking.
3. The forces of nature, including wind, rain, sun, heat, magnetism, gravity, and electricity.

Local Points: Acupressure points located in the area they benefit. See Distal Points.

Lumbar Vertebrae: The last five spinal bones on the lower back above the sacrum.

Lumbosacral Area: The area of the lower back where the lumbar vertebrae join the sacrum.

Medial: Toward the center of the body.

Meditations: Focusing one's attention for developing the spiritual capabilities of the mind.

Meridians: The pathways along which human energy flows through the body, connecting the various acupressure/acupuncture points and the internal organs.

Yin Meridians:

Lung	Lu
Spleen	Sp
Heart	H
Kidney	K
Triple Warmer	TW
Liver	Lv
Conception Vessel	CV

Yang Meridians:

Large Intestine	LI
Stomach	St
Small Intestine	SI
Bladder	B
Pericardium	P
Gall Bladder	GB
Governing Vessel	GV

Metatarsals: The bones between the ankle and toes, on the top of the foot.

Movement Therapy: Using dance and creative movements as a form of self-healing.

Nervous System: The network of nerves that regulates muscular functioning. It influences the coordination of every cell, organ, and system in the body.

Physical Therapy: Neuro-muscular and manipulative re-education techniques for relieving arthritic pain. Chiropractic and osteopathy often use a variety of these joint mobilization techniques.

Pressure Points: Places on the human anatomy with high levels of electrical conductivity. They tend to be located in neuro-muscular junctions, in the joints, and where bones lie close to the skin along a meridian.

Referred Pain: Pain generated in one area of the body, but felt in another.

Sacral: Having to do with the sacrum. (See also Sacrum.)

Sacrum: The flat triangular bone in the lower back at the base of the spine.

Sacroilliac Joints: The two places in the lower back where the sacrum joins the hip bones.

Shiatsu: A Japanese form of acupressure that uses various finger pressure massage techniques on points along the meridians.

Spinal Column: The backbone, composed of a series of bones called vertebrae, which are stacked on top of one another. It protects the spinal cord.

Spinal Cord: The thick cord of nerve tissue of the central nervous system that runs through the spinal column and into the brain.

Spinal Discs: The layer of fibrous connective tissue with small masses of cartilage located between each vertebrae.

Spinal Vertebrae: See Vertebrae.

Thoracic Vertebrae: The twelve spinal vertebrae below the neck in the upper and middle back. See diagram, page 118 .

Vertebrae: The bones of the spinal column through which the spinal cord runs. See Cervical, Thoracic, and Lumbar Vertebrae.

Visualization: A creative process of forming images and thoughts that positively direct one's life.

EXPLANATION OF TERMS

Massage: Use all parts of your hand to smoothly move over the skin, covering the area to stimulate circulation.

Slap: Use the palm side of the fingers to stimulate the area being worked on with a short, quick tempo.

Pound: Make a fist, and keep your wrist loose.

Knead: Gradually grasp the muscles by bringing your fingers toward your thumb, rhythmically squeezing and releasing.

Rub: Briskly move your hand over the surface of the skin in a concentrated area.

Scratch: Use your nails to gently stimulate the surface of the skin.

Press: Use your thumbs, fingers, or the heels of your hands to hold with light to firm pressure.

Squeeze: Firmly grasp hold for several seconds; gradually release.

Roll: Enclose the area with your fingers or hand, and move back and forth in a circular motion.

Rake: Use your fingertips to glide over the surface of the skin, with your fingers comfortably spread and bent to form the shape of a claw.

INDEX

ABOUT THE AUTHOR

Michael Reed Gach is the founder of the Acupressure Institute in Berkeley, California. The Institute is approved by the Board of Registered Nurses and the Department of Education for Vocational Training. Gach received his B.A. in Social Relations from Immaculate Heart College and is currently working on his Ph.D. in Acupressure Health Care at Columbia Pacific University. He holds a community college credential in Health, Physical Care Services, and Related Technologies.

Gach is the author of *The Bum Back Book*, *Acu-Yoga*, and his recent *Greater Energy At Your Fingertips* (Celestial Arts). Over ten years of research enabled Gach to originate a self-help stress management system incorporating acupressure and yoga postures. His *Acu-Yoga* book (published by Japan Publications, distributed by Harper & Row), is in its seventh printing and has been published in German as well as in Spanish.

Michael Reed Gach can be reached by writing to:

Acupressure Institute of America, Inc.
1533 Shattuck Avenue, Dept. 4
Berkeley, CA 94709